MEDICAL INNOVATION AT THE CROSSROADS

VOLUME I

Modern Methods
of
Clinical
Investigation

Annetine C. Gelijns
Editor

Committee on Technological Innovation in Medicine

INSTITUTE OF MEDICINE

NATIONAL ACADEMY PRESS
Washington, D.C. 1990

NATIONAL ACADEMY PRESS • 2101 Constitution Avenue, N.W. • Washington, D.C. 20418

The Institute of Medicine was chartered in 1970 by the National Academy of Sciences to enlist distinguished members of the appropriate professions in the examination of policy matters pertaining to the health of the public. In this, the Institute acts under both the Academy's 1863 congressional charter responsibility to be an advisor to the federal government and its own initiative in identifying issues of medical care, research, and education.

The Committee on Technological Innovation in Medicine was established in 1988 by the Institute of Medicine to design a series of workshops that would (a) provide a more fundamental knowledge of the process by which biomedical research findings are translated into clinical practice, and (b) address opportunities for improving the rationality and efficiency of this process. This volume consists of the proceedings of the first workshop in this series, "Improving the Translation of Research Findings into Clinical Practice: The Potential and Problems of Modern Methods of Clinical Investigation," held on May 3-4, 1989. This workshop and its proceedings were supported by the Howard Hughes Medical Institute and the National Center for Health Services Research of the Department of Health and Human Services (grant 5 RO9 HS055 26 02). The opinions and conclusions expressed here are those of the authors and do not necessarily represent the views of the Howard Hughes Medical Institute, the Department of Health and Human Services, the National Academy of Sciences, or any of their constituent parts.

Library of Congress Cataloging-in-Publication Data

Modern methods of clinical investigation/Annetine C. Gelijns, editor
; Committee on Technological Innovation in Medicine, Institute of
Medicine.
    p. cm. — (Medical innovation at the crossroads ; v. 1)
  Proceedings of a workshop held on May 3-4, 1989, supported by the
Howard Hughes Medical Institute and the National Center for Health
Services Research of the Department of Health and Human Services
(grant 5 RO9 HS055 26 02).
  Includes bibliographical references.
  Includes index.
  ISBN 0-309-04286-0
  1. Medical technology—Evaluation—Congresses. 2. Medical
innovations—Evaluation—Congresses. 3. Medical care—Technological
innovations—Congresses. 4. Meta-analysis—Congresses.
I. Gelijns, Annetine. II. Institute of Medicine (U.S.). Committee
on Technological Innovation in Medicine. III. Howard Hughes Medical
Institute. IV. National Center for Health Services Research.
V. Series.
  [DNLM: 1. Evaluation Studies—congresses. 2. Outcome and Process
Assessment (Health Care)—congresses. 3. Research Design—
congresses. W 20.5 M689 1989]
  R855.2.M63 1990
  610'.72—dc20
  DNLM/DLC
  for Library of Congress   90-6195
                                            CIP

Committee on Technological Innovation in Medicine

Acknowledgments

The Committee on Technological Innovation in Medicine expresses its gratitude to the authors for the high quality of the papers they prepared for this volume. These papers were originally presented at the Institute of Medicine workshop, "Improving the Translation of Research Findings into Clinical Practice: The Potential and Problems of Modern Methods of Clinical Investigation." The committee also recognizes the significant contributions of the moderators, panel discussants, and workshop participants who provided valuable insights into the issues discussed here. Special thanks are due to Paul Friedman, Dean for Academic Personnel at the University of California, San Diego, who prepared a written summary of the workshop discussions that was invaluable in the preparation of this volume. The committee also greatly appreciates the help provided by Frederick Telling, Vice-President for Planning and Policy at Pfizer, Inc. Finally, Edward Edelson is to be thanked for his skillful and expeditious editing of the papers in this volume.

The committee expresses its gratitude to Samuel Thier, President of the Institute of Medicine, for his initiative on behalf of this committee's activities. The committee also is grateful for the substantive and organizational support of Enriqueta Bond, Executive Officer; Ruth Bulger, Director of the Health Sciences Policy Division; Steven Bongard, Director of the Forum on Drug Development; and Wallace Waterfall, Editor for the Institute of Medicine. The workshop and the publication of this volume would not have been possible without Holly Dawkins, who devoted considerable effort to the logistics of the meeting as well as to the preparation and review of several drafts of this manuscript. Cliff Goodman, Director of the Council on Health Care Technology, provided worthy administrative and substantive support of the committee's activities. Finally, we acknowledge a considerable debt to Annetine Gelijns, International Fellow of the Institute of Medicine and principal staff officer to the committee, for her conceptualization of the workshop and the editing of this volume.

The Committee on Technological Innovation in Medicine greatly appreciates the opportunity provided by the Howard Hughes Medical Institute and the National Center for Health Services Research and Technology Assessment (grant HS 055 26) to investigate the process of medical innovation.

GERALD D. LAUBACH
Chair
Committee on Technological
Innovation in Medicine

Preface

GERALD D. LAUBACH

This volume summarizes the first of a series of Institute of Medicine (IOM) workshops whose intent is to critically examine the process by which biomedical research is translated into actual benefits in medical practice.

Contemporary biomedical research has given us a rich harvest of innovation—new pharmaceuticals, biotechnology products, medical devices, and clinical procedures—which in the aggregate essentially define modern, cutting-edge medicine. As always, such success is accompanied by challenges and problems. Some critics believe that certain medical technologies have been adopted too quickly, at the peril of patients or their pocketbooks. As our experience with AIDS has vividly demonstrated, others consider the pace of adoption to be far too slow, unnecessarily depriving patients of desperately needed medical advances. Cost has also become an important concern. The cost of biomedical research and development in general, and clinical investigation in particular, has escalated dramatically over the past two decades.

Because the process of clinical assessment is such a critical determinant of the efficiency, effectiveness, and cost of developing medical technology, the IOM Committee on Technological Innovation in Medicine chose to devote its first workshop to an examination of the status and potential of newer techniques and methods in clinical evaluation. We were further encouraged to make this topic as our lead-off theme by two additional considerations. One of these is the fact that there now exists a considerable variety of relatively new techniques—based on non-traditional statistical concepts, the availability of large medical data bases, and the like—that suggest themselves as useful adjuncts to the process of clinical evaluation. But the appropriate application and ultimate power and usefulness of these methods are not entirely clear.

The second consideration underlying our choice is the notable broadening of the questions that are being asked of clinical evaluation. Society now seeks information about new biomedical technologies that goes beyond the traditional issues of safety and efficacy. In many cases, for example, a new pharmaceutical might be appropriately evaluated not only against existing drugs for the same condition but also against alternative medical devices or procedures. Increasingly, we seek information about the longer-term impact of a medical intervention as it expresses itself in the real world of everyday clinical practice, as contrasted with the more focused and nearly ideal setting characteristic of controlled clinical trials. We ask, and indeed should ask, questions about rare and idiosyncratic consequences of medical interventions—questions that can only be practically answered through access to data bases accumulated after very large numbers of patient exposures. Here, again, newer methodologies present themselves as powerful additions to the more traditional techniques.

Finally, the United States currently has a patchwork process of technology transfer in biomedicine. In particular, there is a concern that regulatory approaches developed over the past four decades may not be evolving suitably to keep up with the exponential growth in biomedical knowledge, more recent developments in the clinical evaluative sciences, and the changing economics of health care. Our regulatory system has grown more or less haphazardly, and one of its most notable features is a remarkable asymmetry across the different classes of technology. A new drug must undergo long and stringent testing to be approved for a given medical indication. But whereas this process of drug evaluation is closely regulated, the adoption of new clinical procedures essentially falls outside the regulatory scope—unless the procedure should happen to use a new instrument, in which case regulatory agencies become involved to a limited degree, depending on the nature of the device. Powerful forces in contemporary health policy, not least the concern about marked and inexplicable regional variations in medical practice, seem to be pressing toward a more consistent and even-handed assessment of all kinds of medical technology, including comparisons of alternative modalities of management for a given medical condition. The optimum approach and methodology for accomplishing this challenging task are yet to be defined.

The papers presented at this workshop essentially address two questions about clinical evaluation: How well are we doing it? How can we improve it? They provide a rich variety of answers and other key insights, with examples drawn from clinical practice, evaluations, and statistical methodology. The clear sense that emerges is that we can do better, and that the tools for improvement are at hand.

The committee held its second workshop in December 1989. It explored and analyzed the changing economics of technological innovation in medicine, drawing on experience in the United States, Europe, and Japan. At present, two additional workshops on issues in medical innovation are being organized. Together, this series of workshops will offer a coherent body of study and analysis for improving our understanding of medical innovation. It is our hope that this work will encourage a more rational and efficient transfer of biomedical research findings into direct patient care.

Contents

List of Tables and Figures

TABLES

xiii

FIGURES

List of Abbreviations

AIDS	Acquired Immune Deficiency Syndrome
AUA	American Urological Association
BPH	Benign Prostatic Hyperplasia
CABG	Coronary Artery Bypass Grafting
CON	Certificate of Need
CSM	Committee on Safety of Medicines (United Kingdom)
DES	Diethylstilbestrol
DSRU	Drug Safety Research Unit (United Kingdom)
FDA	Food and Drug Administration
FD&CA	Food, Drug, and Cosmetics Act
GAO	General Accounting Office
GMP	Good Manufacturing Practices
HCFA	Health Care Financing Administration
IDE	Investigational Device Exemption
IMS	Intercontinental Medical Statistics Limited
IND	Investigational New Drug
IOM	Institute of Medicine
IRB	Institutional Review Board
MRI	Magnetic Resonance Imaging
NCE	New Chemical Entity
NDA	New Drug Application
NHLBI	National Heart, Lung, and Blood Institute
NIH	National Institutes of Health
NSAIDs	Non-steroidal Anti-inflammatory Drugs
PEM	Prescription-Event Monitoring (United Kingdom)

PMA	Pre-marketing Application for Devices
PMS	Post-marketing Surveillance
POARP	Patient Outcomes Assessment Research Program
PPA	Prescription Pricing Authority (United Kingdom)
PPS	Prospective Payment System
PTCA	Percutaneous Transluminal Coronary Angioplasty
R&D	Research and Development
RCT	Randomized Controlled Clinical Trial
ROC	Receiver Operating Characteristic
t-PA	Tissue Plasminogen Activator
TURP	Transurethral Resection of the Prostate

1

Medical Technology Development: An Introduction to the Innovation-Evaluation Nexus

ANNETINE C. GELIJNS and SAMUEL O. THIER

The increase in fundamental knowledge concerning human health and the mechanisms of disease has been so rapid during the second half of this century that we have often been described as living in a time of biological revolution. In the spirit of Francis Bacon, who observed that the true essence of progress is in the application of scientific knowledge for enhancing the human condition, our society for the past several decades has valued biomedical innovation and its promise of improving the management of health and disease. Rapid advances in biomedical research have indeed stimulated the development of numerous efficacious medical technologies, but their translation into clinical use has raised complex medical, economic, and social issues. The emergence of these issues—as illustrated by the development of new aquired immune deficiency syndrome (AIDS) drugs—is spurring new interest in medical innovation: how it occurs, what can be expected of it, and how it might be improved.

Technological innovation in medicine covers the wide range of events by which a new medical technology is discovered or invented, developed, and disseminated into health care. One of the most vulnerable links in this innovation chain today is the development phase, the "D" of R&D, in which research findings are brought into clinical practice. More specifically, medical technology development can be defined as a multi-stage process through which a new biological or chemical agent, prototype medical device, or clinical procedure is technically modified and clinically evaluated until it is considered ready for general use. Although this definition suggests an organized and systematic process, much developmental activity actually occurs in a non-orderly fashion in everyday clinical practice.

1

Among the many factors influencing development, the criteria and methods of clinical evaluation have become increasingly important determinants of how—and indeed whether—new medical technologies are developed. This first volume of the Institute of Medicine (IOM) Committee on Technological Innovation in Medicine focuses on the interplay between strategies for clinical evaluation and the development of new drugs, devices, and clinical procedures.

PUTTING CLINICAL EVALUATION IN CONTEXT

Two major considerations influenced the selection of the theme of this volume. The first is the emergence of widespread concern over the way in which new medical technologies are evaluated clinically during the development process.[1] For example, the development of drugs for life-threatening diseases has become the subject of extensive reporting in the professional literature and the daily press, as well as a matter of serious policy debate. A key issue is whether the pre-marketing evaluative requirements governing drug development are sufficiently flexible or are interpreted flexibly enough in the case of drugs for fatal diseases such as cancer or AIDS. For example, one might question whether and when intermediate endpoints, instead of survival, should be evaluated in pre-approval trials. The Food, Drug, and Cosmetic Act allows considerable latitude for subjective interpretation of the terms "safety" and "effectiveness" in determining the acceptable risk-benefit ratio for a marketing approval decision.[2] But because of social and political pressures to reduce the risk to essentially zero, pre-marketing requirements have become increasingly detailed over time. Although the resulting system has provided important information on the efficacy and safety of new drugs, it has also considerably lengthened the pre-marketing development process. Moreover, despite this increase, there are clearly no "zero-risk" approval decisions. For example, the detection of delayed or rare (less than 1:10,000) adverse effects would require extremely long periods of testing or the exposure of many thousands of patients. Furthermore, valuable therapeutic information on the risks and benefits of a new drug may emerge only *after* its diffusion into the often messy environment of general use. For instance, in the period 1982-1986, six newly approved drugs were withdrawn shortly after introduction and five others required substantial relabeling, despite

---

[1] This concern is also evident regarding the economic evaluation of new technologies during their development. This issue will be the subject of a subsequent publication, and thus will not be further discussed in this volume.

[2] Effectiveness refers to the probability of benefits under average conditions of use, and efficacy refers to this under ideal conditions of use. Although the law uses the term effectiveness, the approval decision is made on the basis of efficacy information. This paper will therefore use the term efficacy in the context of pre-marketing clinical investigations, that is, to refer to testing under ideal conditions of use.

rigorous pre-marketing evaluation (1). A classic example of side effects that may be hard to detect in the carefully controlled setting of pre-approval trials is the acute hypertension induced by the antidepressant tranylcypromine if the patient happens to eat a particular kind of cheese. The traditional response to the realization that taking drugs may be a risky business has been to increase pre-marketing requirements for clinical evaluation. It is now timely to ask whether this strategy will remain appropriate or whether a point of diminishing returns has been reached, and if a shift in emphasis toward obtaining information in the post-marketing clinical setting would not be more appropriate.

A different issue is concern about the adequacy of the evidence underlying development and dissemination of clinical procedures into health care (2). For example, extracranial-intracranial vascular bypass surgery for stroke was first tried in human beings in 1967; the procedure underwent rapid diffusion during the 1970s, but was only recently reported ineffective in preventing cerebral ischemia in patients with atherosclerotic disease of the carotid and middle cerebral arteries (3). At a national level, the considerable geographic variations in the use of certain clinical procedures may largely be explained by insufficient evidence about their diagnostic, therapeutic, and ultimate health effects (4). The consequences of such variations for the quality of medical care and the cost-effective use of resources hardly need further explanation, and an argument for more systematic evaluation of clinical procedures has been made repeatedly. Important questions, however, remain as to what evidence should be collected and by what methods during the various stages of the development process. For example, when during the development of a new surgical procedure should a randomized controlled clinical trial be initiated? What are the strengths and weaknesses of modern epidemiological methods during the evolution of new clinical procedures? Given the increasing importance of quality of life as an endpoint in medical care, how do we obtain a more systematic understanding of patient preferences about different health outcomes? And which policy and institutional mechanisms can assure that adequate clinical studies of new procedures are indeed undertaken? These issues, which concern the scientific basis for decisions during development, need to be addressed urgently.

The second consideration for focusing on the interplay between clinical evaluation and technology development concerns the rapid progress occurring in the art and science of clinical evaluation today. Since its inception in the early 1950s, the randomized controlled clinical trial (RCT) has been accepted as an extremely powerful tool for assessing the efficacy of new drugs and biologicals. However, it has also become clear that RCTs are not necessarily practical or feasible for answering all clinical questions. Therefore, a variety of other methods, such as non-randomized trials or observational methods, have been adopted to provide complementary information. Traditionally, these methods were regarded as weaker than RCTs for clinical evaluation. Recent methodological advances, such as the use of non-classical statistics and the ability to link large-scale automated data bases for analysis (e.g., those of health insurance networks and hospitals), are strengthening these approaches. In addition, methods for synthesizing the evidence that results both from experimental and observational studies are being improved. The IOM Committee on Technological Innovation in Medicine observed that these methods may well provide an opportunity to address some of the concerns mentioned above. Although these methods are conceptually appealing, there are important questions as to their strengths and weaknesses and the quality of the evidence they provide.

In view of these considerations, it seemed timely to publish a volume of papers analyzing the validity of these modern methods of clinical investigation and asking if and how their systematic application could improve the technology development process. Before addressing some of the points made by the various authors, a more complete picture is needed of current shortcomings in the clinical evaluation of new medical technologies. The following section will explore some of these shortcomings, using the development of specific pharmacological, surgical, and medical device technologies for the treatment of stable angina pectoris as a case example.

ISSUES IN INNOVATION AND EVALUATION: THE CASE OF STABLE ANGINA PECTORIS

Beta-Blockers

In the late 1950s, Slater and Powell at Eli Lilly serendipitously discovered the pharmaceutical compound dichloroisoproterenol while developing long-acting bronchodilators (5). This compound was found to have beta-adrenergic blockade activity, but also had partial agonist (sympathomimetic) activity; its development was not pursued. At the same time James Black—a 1988 Nobel laureate for physiology or medicine—hypothesized that blocking the beta-adrenergic receptors would diminish the heart's demand for oxygen, providing relief for angina sufferers. He saw the clinical potential of dichloroisoproterenol, and with his colleagues at Imperial Chemical Industries (ICI) started to synthesize its analogues. The first of these compounds to be tested in humans, pronethalol, had a beneficial effect on angina in Phase I trials (6). In a full-scale clinical trial, however, it induced such side effects as nausea, vomiting, and light-headedness. When long-term toxicity tests in animals revealed that it might also be carcinogenic, its development was discontinued. Subsequently, propranolol was synthesized and found to be free of both the agonist activity of dichloroisoproterenol and the side effects of pronethalol (7).[3] It became the first beta-adrenergic antagonist to be marketed in the United Kingdom in 1965 (see Figure 1.1).

---

[3]Koppe of Boehringer Ingelheim synthesized propanolol shortly before pronethalol was discovered. However, its clinical potential was not recognized at the time, and no patent was filed.

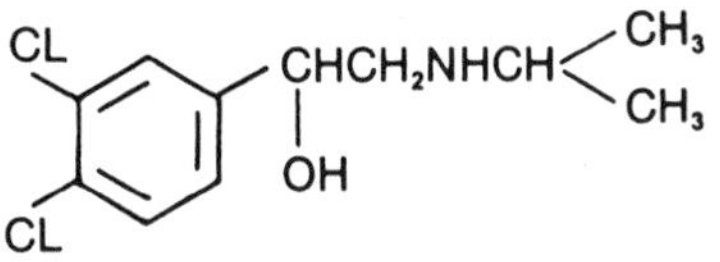

Dichloroisoproterenol

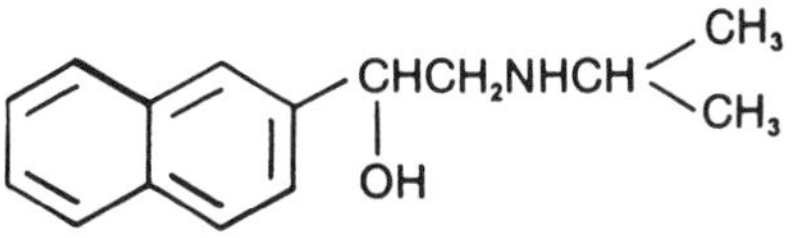

Pronethalol

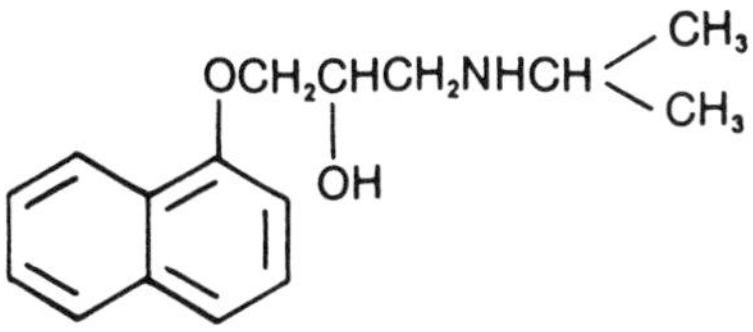

Propranolol

FIGURE 1.1 Small chemical differences but large clinical differences.

In subsequent years, structural analogues of propranolol were introduced on the basis of systematic animal testing and clinical evaluation. These early beta-blockers acted on all beta-adrenergic receptors, which was troublesome for asthmatics. In 1966, Dunlop and Shanks of ICI discovered an analogue that acted selectively on heart receptors (8). This compound was marketed in 1970 in the United Kingdom as practolol, for use by asthmatic patients. In spite of rigorous pre-marketing evaluation, practolol was found to cause very serious side effects, including blindness, in day-to-day clinical practice. Although the incidence of these events was high—1:500—and the events emerged shortly after widespread use began, it took a year or more, during which 100,000 or more patients were treated, before the first voluntary reports reached the Committee on Safety of Medicines and the drug was withdrawn.

As a result of the practolol incident, there was a growing awareness that the system of adverse effect reporting alone, however valuable for the detection of very rare effects, was insufficient for optimal clinical and regulatory decision making. In the United Kingdom, Inman established the Prescription-Event Monitoring Scheme, which tracks the performance of all new chemical entities in clinical practice, to speed the early detection and analysis of adverse events (see Chapter 6). Such monitoring also can facilitate the earlier detection and analysis of benefits; following their introduction into practice, beta-blockers were found to be of potential value in a wide variety of cardiac and non-cardiac conditions. They now are used for more than 20 medical conditions, including hypertension, myocardial infarction, anxiety, and alcoholism (9). Because drugs, once marketed, are subject to empirical innovation and the regulatory system is designed not to interfere with the practice of medicine, the clinical evidence supporting drug use for specific conditions can be quite variable. By

1987, for example, the Food and Drug Administration (FDA) had approved only eight of the many conditions for which beta-blockers are used. Although industrial, governmental, and academic investment in post-marketing pharmaceutical research is increasing, this area remains relatively underdeveloped.

Coronary Artery Bypass Grafting

The development of surgical techniques for angina pectoris presents quite a different picture. The evolution of such surgery can be traced to the turn of the century when cardiac denervation was proposed as a treatment for the crippling pain associated with the disease (10). In the decades preceding the first clinical application of coronary artery bypass grafting (CABG), many new surgical techniques were developed by surgical schools in a variety of countries. Often these procedures coexisted for years, only to be discarded later because of inadequate efficacy or unacceptable side effects. As Effler argues, the earliest surgical development was based on a bad premise: treatment preceded diagnosis (11). It is only with the introduction of Mason Sones's arteriography in 1958 that the success of surgery in terms of graft patency could be validated objectively, and rational patient selection criteria established. Rene Favaloro at the Cleveland Clinic is generally credited with the first report on coronary artery bypass surgery using a saphenous vein graft in 1968 (12). Following the initial discussion of the new procedure at conferences and in the literature, it underwent rapid diffusion and further incremental development. Clinical circumstances favored swift acceptance of the operation: the condition is life-threatening and decreases quality of life, especially for those unresponsive to drug treatment; the operation made sense anatomically and physiologically; and from the outset it seemed very effective in the relief of disabling angina (13). The feeling that the procedure was rational and the fact that the technical aspects of the procedure were still evolving led to a situation in which randomized studies were not carried out; the surgical innovators and those who followed them felt it was too early for an RCT. In the first years there were many publications on graft patency, mortality, and relief of angina, all on the basis of uncontrolled clinical series. With increasing surgical experience and incremental improvements in surgical technique, mortality rates decreased considerably. By 1972-1973, many felt CABG had become the treatment of choice for patients with severe stable angina, and that it was thus too late to carry out RCTs (13). Although there was no dispute about the new procedure's efficacy in relieving the pain of angina, doubt remained about its effect on survival. Three large multicenter RCTs were initiated during the 1970s to analyze the effect on life expectancy: the Veterans Administration (VA) trial, the European Cooperative Surgery Study, and the Coronary Artery Surgery Study (CASS) (14-16). At the end of the 1970s these trials provided valuable evidence on the safety and efficacy of CABG in specific patient groups, and follow-up results on long-term safety and efficacy were published during the 1980s (17,18).

Although these trials made an important contribution to our knowledge base, two major questions emerge from the above pattern of innovation and evaluation. The trials provided their initial information on safety and efficacy 10 years after the procedure had first been used in clinical practice. During that decade, clinical decision making had to depend to a large extent on anecdotal evidence. As Preston remarks when he argues for encouragement of surgical innovation but questions the process of development itself: "Can the profession afford yet another cycle of unrecognized experimentation, widespread application without validation of benefit, immense economic and professional gratification, gradual disillusionment, and ultimate abandonment in favor of the next 'new' operation?" (10). In other words, the question is whether establishing a mechanism to systematically initiate and coordinate surgical trials on the basis of early clinical experience (analogous to Phase I drug trials) could have expedited the design and implementation of CABG trials.[4]

The other question is whether trial results carried out a decade ago can still be considered valid today. During these years, the indications for CABG have widened to include unstable angina, myocardial infarction, and minimal angina pectoris. Hlatky et al., for example, compared the patient population in the cardiovascular disease data base at Duke University with the patients enrolled in the above-mentioned RCTs (19). They found that only 13 percent met the criteria for the VA trial, 8 percent met the eligibility criteria for the European study, and 4 percent met those for the CASS. In addition to such changes in patient indications, surgical techniques have also undergone further development. For example, internal mammary arteries have recently been found to have a much higher long-term patency rate than saphenous vein grafts (20). In the three RCTs, however, internal mammary arteries were used in only a very small number of cases. These examples illustrate the need for long-term surveillance of new procedures as they evolve in everyday clinical practice.

PTCA Catheter Equipment

In 1977, Andreas Gruentzig at the University of Zurich performed the first clinical percutaneous transluminal coronary angioplasty (PTCA) procedure as an alternative to coronary artery bypass surgery (21). With the firm Schneider-

---

[4]For example, although the use of CABG in humans was first reported in 1968, the VA trial in 1972 originally set out to evaluate the much earlier developed Vineberg procedure. Only after some time did it shift its resources to CABG. If there had been a mechanism to monitor surgical development, this delay could perhaps have been prevented.

Medintag, he developed a flexible double-lumen dilation catheter with a balloon that could be inflated to compress the deposits that block an artery. In 1979, Gruentzig reported on his first 50 patients in *The New England Journal of Medicine* and concluded that his results were "preliminary." More information and follow-up data are needed before coronary angioplasty can be accepted as one form of treatment for coronary-artery disease. However, the results in patients with single-vessel disease are sufficiently good to make the procedure acceptable for prospective randomized trials. Such trials are clearly needed if we are to evaluate the efficacy of this new technique as compared with current medical and surgical techniques" (22). Among cardiologists, however, there was a strong feeling that comparative trials of PTCA and medical or surgical therapy should be delayed until the technology had evolved and the learning curves were established. Thus, the National Heart, Lung, and Blood Institute established an international voluntary registry in 1979 to monitor the safety and effectiveness of PTCA.

Under the newly established medical device amendments to the Food, Drug, and Cosmetics Law, the first balloon dilation catheter was approved for marketing in the United States by the FDA in 1980 (23). To date, nine dilation catheter systems have undergone full pre-marketing safety and efficacy review by the FDA. All were approved not on the basis of RCTs, but on the basis of comparing the results of clinical series with those of other marketed PTCA devices or registry data. Because the PTCA market is very competitive, new modifications emerge almost every month and any product can be outdated within 6 to 12 months (24). These incremental improvements do not require full FDA review but are approved under so-called supplemental pre-marketing approval decisions. In addition to rapid technological change, patient selection criteria are also changing considerably. PTCA was initially used predominantly in discrete noncalcified single-vessel lesions, but it is now being applied in disease affecting multiple vessels and where there are multiple lesions in the same vessel, as well as in unstable angina and acute infarction. The National Institutes of Health (NIH) registry data have been extremely valuable in monitoring these changes in technology and application, as well as their effects on effectiveness and safety. Despite these data, however, there is still no conclusive evidence on the comparative efficacy and safety of PTCA versus medical treatment in single vessel disease, and of PTCA versus CABG in multivessel disease. Randomized controlled clinical trials are clearly overdue. In 1987, the NIH and the VA decided to support three such clinical trials; their results, however, are not expected until the early 1990s to mid-1990s.

Evaluative Shortcomings in Technology Development

The example of stable angina pectoris refutes a popular belief, which holds technology development to be a linear progression from bench to bedside. Surgical innovation often occurs in a decentralized environment with numerous surgical schools trying to find a solution to a particular problem in day-to-day practice. Drugs and devices are also subject to further development in clinical practice. New indications can be revealed in practice, as illustrated by the off-label use of beta-blockers. Also, early clinical experience with a new product may provide impetus to the development of improved products. For example, due to such feedback PTCA catheters have been miniaturized, made more flexible, and given improved angiographic visibility. A more realistic picture of technology development, in which development and diffusion are highly interactive and partially overlap, is the basis for discussing shortcomings in today's strategies for clinical evaluation.

The often inadequate conceptualization in health sciences policy of innovation as linear and sequential has contributed to a system of clinical investigation with major emphasis on providing safety and efficacy information prior to a technology's diffusion. However, as the angina pectoris case illustrates, certain information on the risks and benefits of a technology may emerge only after its diffusion into general use. Furthermore, much developmental activity occurs not before but *during* everyday practice; consider, for instance, changes in surgical technique or in patient indications. Evaluative strategies, however, have rarely attempted to provide information on the effectiveness and long-term safety of technologies as they evolve in normal, uncontrolled, daily medical life.

In addition, the angina pectoris example reveals a remarkable asymmetry in the existing strategies for providing safety and efficacy information: drugs undergo rigorous clinical testing before their introduction into general use, clinical procedures are still assessed mainly in an *ad hoc* fashion, and evaluations of new medical devices are somewhere in between. For example, a randomized trial was initiated a few weeks after the initial testing of a beta-blocker in humans, but it took five years before the first RCT was initiated for CABG. From a historical perspective, differences in the nature of innovation among drugs, devices, and procedures have contributed to different types of regulatory approaches, which in turn have contributed to this imbalance in safety and efficacy information (see Appendix A). Clinical and other health care decisions, however, require comparable information first on the safety and efficacy of a new technology, and then on its effectiveness. Moreover, because the management of clinical conditions such as stable angina increasingly requires choices among alternative diagnostic and therapeutic options, information is also needed on the relative effectiveness and safety of all the various technological alternatives. There are few assessments that provide this kind of information, and these shortcomings in evaluative strategies have been detrimental to a rational and efficient transfer of biomedical research findings into clinical practice.

IMPROVING THE INNOVATION-EVALUATION NEXUS

A major premise of this volume is that we need a more balanced assessment strategy that depends on an adequate model of the development phase within the innovation continuum. The papers in this volume deal with the design and implementation of such a strategy, and address three major issues: (1) What kinds of clinical evidence or endpoints should be evaluated during what stage of the development process? (2) What is the role of observational methods relative to experimental methods (including RCTs) in providing this evidence, and what is the role of methods for synthesizing primary clinical data? (3) What policy mechanisms would ensure that adequate clinical evidence is a major decision-making factor during the development phase of the innovation process?

The Selection of Endpoints in Evaluative Research

A spectrum of relevant endpoints, ranging from physiological or anatomical parameters to mortality, morbidity, health status, functional status, and quality of life, can be evaluated during the development process. The notion of what constitutes valid endpoints is in continual flux. Because many therapeutic agents for today's chronic degenerative diseases treat only symptoms, improvements in functional status, health status, and quality of life are increasingly important endpoints in clinical evaluation. However, Marilyn Bergner in this volume asserts that the inclusion of health status or quality of life considerations in clinical trials is often an afterthought. She argues for a broader approach, especially regarding quality of life, and the inclusion of measures that are reliable and well-validated in clinical trials.

Kenneth Melmon contends that the different participants in the development process—those in industry, regulatory agencies, and clinical research and practice—require different kinds of evidence as a basis for their decision making. This is well illustrated, for example, by the differences in information needed for regulatory decisions as distinct from clinical decisions. The marketing approval decision requires evidence of a new technology's safety and efficacy, but post-marketing regulatory decisions require evidence on its long-term safety in everyday clinical practice. Clinical decisions, however, also require information on effectiveness, and if various technological alternatives are involved in the management of a clinical condition, on *relative* effectiveness. Furthermore, insight is needed into patient preferences for the health benefits and risks associated with these options.

In the context of regulatory approval decisions, considerable uncertainty exists over the role of intermediate endpoints as surrogates for such clinical endpoints as mortality, morbidity, disability, and quality of life. In some cases the FDA has accepted intermediate endpoints, such as lowered blood pressure with the use of anti-hypertensives. But the value of surrogate endpoints is in dispute for matters such as tissue plasminogen activator, erythropoietin, and cancer chemotherapy. As John Bunker illustrates, the acceptability of these endpoints is affected by such factors as the lethality of the disease, the availability of alternative technologies, the length of time before clinical results will be known, and the strength of the relationship between intermediate endpoints and the patient outcomes of disease treatment. In those cases where intermediate endpoints are appropriate, regulatory acceptance can be increased by systematic follow-up of clinical endpoints in the post-marketing setting.

Several authors in this volume emphasize the need to improve monitoring of outcomes in "real world" clinical practice. Chapter 2 underlines the need to include all-cause outcomes, in addition to disease-specific outcomes, in these studies. For example, some have questioned whether the decrease in cardiac mortality associated with lowering blood cholesterol may be offset by an increase in cancer mortality. To date, the concept of offsetting risks and benefits in innovation remains weak and often is not taken sufficiently into account.

The Selection of Methods for Clinical Investigation

A variety of experimental and observational methods can provide the needed evidence. As mentioned, the RCT is generally regarded as the statistically most powerful method for determining pharmaceutical efficacy in pre-marketing evaluations. During the development of devices and clinical procedures, some real conceptual, practical, and ethical difficulties may exist regarding the use of RCTs, and efficacy evaluation will need to depend on other adequately controlled study designs. John Wennberg, for example, argues that randomization may be unethical when alternative treatment modalities are being developed to increase quality of life, if different interventions are associated with very variable risks and benefits. In this situation, assignment according to patient preferences may be an ethically unavoidable imperative. The value of patient preference trials depends on our ability to distinguish therapeutic effects from effects of preference, placebo, and compliance. Today this understanding is not available, but an innovative research proposal to start disentangling these effects is described in Chapter 4.

Following randomized or otherwise well-controlled safety and efficacy trials, long-term surveillance should be undertaken of the safety and effectiveness of new technologies in actual use. The emphasis in this volume is on the strengths and weaknesses of observational methods, and their role in providing such information. With regard to drugs, William Inman discusses the United

Kingdom's Prescription-Event Monitoring System. Using prescription-based cohorts as a starting point, this system actively solicits responses from physicians about patient events (which are very different from suspected adverse effects). In essence, this system links pharmacy records with medical record data bases. Similarly, the FDA, industry, and academia are increasingly investing in the use of Medicaid and other medical record linkage data bases for pharmaco-epidemiological research. Given the increased availability of large-scale automated data bases, the possibilities of inexpensive monitoring of health outcomes are appealing. Leslie and Noralou Roos, Fisher, and Bubolz describe the strengths and weaknesses of health insurance data bases, and discuss how combining administrative and clinical data bases could compensate for some weaknesses. The discussion of the benign prostatic hyperplasia assessment, which compares different surgical techniques and watchful waiting, exemplifies the complementary role of observational methods and experimental methods during the development process.

In addition to methods for primary data analysis, this volume discusses methods for synthesizing existing data and the opportunity they may provide for improving regulatory, industrial, and clinical decision making. If we are to improve clinical decision making, decision analysis is an important tool. As Albert Mulley explains, its value is in the synthesis of the results of both experimental and observational studies, and the distinction it makes between matters of fact—as provided by evaluative research—and value judgments inherent in the use of a technology (for instance, variability in patients' preferences). As such, decision analysis defines uncertainties and demonstrates specific needs for further clinical investigation. Meta-analysis is becoming an important new tool for improving the aggregation of experimental and observational information for decision making purposes, including regulatory decisions. In this respect one will read with interest Stephen Thacker's discussion of meta-analysis techniques based on classical statistics, and David Eddy's discussion of Bayesian statistics. Eddy reviews the existing spectrum of methods, ranging from anecdotal evidence to large-scale RCTs, that can provide clinical evidence during the development process. He asserts that all these methods provide information on the magnitude of risks and benefits, and on the extent of uncertainty in these estimates. The logistics, costs, and time needed for the various study designs differ considerably. In addition, each of these methods is subject to different types of bias that affect its internal and external validity. Because of the complexity of choosing acceptable methods for particular kinds of decisions, decision makers generally apply simple heuristics to determine if a particular study design is acceptable or not. However, these heuristics often do not take into account that different study designs may provide complementary evidence. Furthermore, in view of widespread use of the weaker methods of evaluation and recognizing that decision making often depends on less than perfect information, efforts to improve these methods can be expected to have a substantial impact on enhancing the transfer of biomedical research findings into practice.

Eddy describes a methodological approach that identifies the biases inherent in particular studies, estimates their magnitude, and adjusts the results for these biases. Implementation of this approach would enhance the reliability of various evaluative methods that form the basis of developmental decision making.

Policy Mechanisms for Improving Developmental Decision Making

In the aggregate, this volume reflects on the evaluative shortcomings in the present-day development of drugs, devices, and clinical procedures and argues for a more balanced assessment strategy that provides comparable information on the relevant outcomes for *all* technologies. Recent advances in the art and science of clinical evaluation open up new opportunities for providing this evidence. The major question now remains how to ensure their appropriate application without unduly hampering innovation.

What incentives would encourage increased support of post-marketing research for drugs and devices? This research could provide information on their effectiveness and long-term safety for approved indications, as well as a means for monitoring the emergence of new indications of use. In our opinion, such a change can be effected without modification of the Food, Drug, and Cosmetics Act. Powerful demand and supply factors are stimulating investment in this kind of evaluative research. In today's health care environment, for example, there is an increasing demand for relative effectiveness and long-term safety information by health care professionals and third-party payers, and a growing recognition—from an economic point of view—of the marketing advantages that may accrue if such benefits can be demonstrated. On the supply side, rapid advances in methods for clinical investigation are allowing this information to be provided more reliably and efficiently. This is important in the case of drugs, because the effective patent life for new drugs has decreased considerably over time and the industry is not likely to invest in post-marketing research that provides outcomes information only after the drug has turned generic. The industrial incentive to invest in systematic Phase IV outcomes research would, of course, increase if such investment meant that the time spent in pre-approval evaluations could be shortened.

With regard to procedures, a systematic approach toward providing both "pre-marketing" and "post-marketing" information is needed. We do not wish to imply that the establishment of a federal regulatory system governing the development of procedures is needed or probably would even be effective, especially in view of the decentralized and incremental nature of development. One appealing non-regulatory model for improvement of the innovation-evaluation nexus can be found in the outcomes initiative. It tends to focus on clinical conditions instead of individual technologies, and it provides comparative assessment information on the various technological alternatives. It also includes a diverse spectrum of endpoints, and employs both experimental and observational methods. This initiative would provide a means for early identification of the (incremental) development of procedures in a decentralized environment. On the basis of such information, clinical trials could then be initiated as appropriate. The systematic use of observational methods for monitoring actual performance of new procedures in clinical practice would also allow earlier detection of their long-term safety and effectiveness in everyday use. Moreover, as the focus is on the management of clinical conditions, this initiative will at the same time monitor the long-term effectiveness and safety of the drugs or devices involved.

Federal support for this kind of evaluative research has recently increased. For example, support of outcomes research is a critical part of the congressional mandate to the newly established Agency for Health Care Policy and Research. Drug and device manufacturers can also be expected to take interest in helping fund this initiative as a way of providing relative safety and effectiveness information on their new products. However, if the stronger financial sectors of our health care system (the drug industry, for instance, invests roughly $6.5 billion in R&D in the United States) were to share the financial burden of performing evaluations of clinical procedures, their involvement could pose conflicts of interest. It therefore seems timely to explore acceptable models of private-public cooperation in funding this kind of clinical investigation.

In conclusion, a more rational and efficient development stage in the innovation process will require stronger and new kinds of alliances in evaluative research among the various participants: those who develop new technologies; those who improve and apply the science and tools of evaluation; and those who use the resulting information for regulatory approval, reimbursement, or clinical decisions. It will also require a willingness to explore and debate the often complementary value of various evaluative methods for improving developmental decision making. We hope this volume, the first in a series on issues in medical innovation, will contribute to such a debate.

REFERENCES

1. Wiener H. Problems in the assessment of side effects of new drugs. (photocopy). New York.
2. Eddy DM, Billings J. The quality of medical evidence: Implications for quality of care. Health Affairs 1988;Spring:20–32.
3. EC/IC Bypass Study Group. Failure of extracranial-intracranial bypass to reduce the risk of ischemic stroke. New England Journal of Medicine 1985;313:1191–1200.
4. Wennberg JE. Improving the medical decision making process. Health Affairs 1988;Spring:99–106.
5. Powell EE, Slater IH. Blocking inhibitory adrenergic receptors by a dichloro analog of isoproterenol. Journal of Pharmacology and Experimental Therapeutics 1958;122:480–488.
6. Black JW, Stephenson JS. Pharmacology of a new adrenergic beta-receptor-blocking compound (netholide). Lancet 1962;2:311–314.

7. Black JW, Crowther AF, Shanks RG, Smith LH, Dornhorst AC. A new adrenergic beta receptor antagonist. Lancet 1964;1:1080–1081.

8. Sneader W. Drug Discovery: The Evolution of Modern Medicines. Chichester, U.K.: John Wiley & Sons, 1985.

9. Frishman WH. Clinical differences between beta-adrenergic agents: Implications for therapeutic substitution. American Heart Journal 1987;113:1190–1198.

10. Preston TA. Historical development of operations for coronary artery disease. Chapter 2 in Coronary Artery Surgery: A Critical Review. New York: Raven Press, 1977.

11. Effler DB. Myocardial revascularization surgery since 1945 A.D.: Its evolution and its impact. The Journal of Thoracic and Cardiovascular Surgery 1972; 72:823–828.

12. Favaloro RG. Saphenous vein autograft replacement of severe segmental coronary artery occlusion: Operative technique. Annals of Thoracic Surgery 1968;5:334–339.

13. Bunker JP, Hinkley D, McDermott WV. Surgical innovation and its evaluation. Science 1978;200:937–941.

14. Murphy ML, Hultgren HN, Detrec Thomsen J, Taharo T, and participants of the Veterans Administration Cooperative Study. Treatment of chronic stable angina. A preliminary report of survival data of the randomized Veterans Administration cooperative study. New England Journal of Medicine 1977;297:621–627.

15. European Coronary Surgery Study Group. Long-term results of prospective randomized study of coronary artery bypass surgery in stable angina pectoris. Lancet 1982; 2:1173-1180.

16. Coronary Artery Surgery Study (CASS) principal investigators and their associates. A randomized trial of coronary artery bypass surgery: Survival data. Circulation 1983;68:939–950.

17. The Veterans Administration Coronary Artery Bypass Surgery Cooperative Study Group. Eleven-year survival in the Veterans Administration randomized trial of coronary bypass surgery for stable angina. New England Journal of Medicine 1984; 311:1333–1339.

18. Varnauskas E and the European Coronary Surgery Study Group. Twelve-year follow-up of survival in the randomized European coronary surgery study. New England Journal of Medicine 1988;319:332–337.

19. Hlatky MA, Leek L, Harrel FE, Califf RM, Pryor DB, Marck DB, Rosatti RA. Tying clinical research to patient care by use of an observational database. Statistics in Medicine 1984;3:375–384.

20. Loop FD, Lytle BW, Cosgrove PM et al. Influence of the internal mammary artery graft on 10-year survival and other cardiac events. New England Journal of Medicine 1986;314:1–6.

21. Gruentzig A. Transluminal dilation of coronary-artery stenosis. Lancet 1978;1:263.

22. Gruentzig A, Senning A, Siegenthaler WE. Non-operative dilatation of coronary-artery stenosis: Per-cutaneous transluminal coronary angioplasty. New England Journal of Medicine 1979;301:61–68.

23. USCI Division of CR Bard, Inc. Summary of safety and effectiveness for the USCI Gruentzig Dilaca Coronary Artery Balloon Catheter. Rockville 1980.

24. Topol EJ, Myler RK, Stertzer SH. Selection of dilatation catheter hardware for PTCA-1985. Catheterization and Cardiovascular Diagnosis 1985;11:629–637.

2

The Selection of Endpoints in Evaluative Research

JOHN P. BUNKER

Having repeatedly urged that we make a greater investment in the evaluation of medical technologies, it is perhaps only fitting that I discuss the endpoints one should address during the various stages of the development process, and when one might rely on intermediate endpoints as surrogates for clinical endpoints. I will consider condition-specific mortality versus all-cause mortality, and—where mortality is not a central issue—condition-specific outcomes versus all-cause outcomes. I will also address the underlying issue of risks and benefits; that is, the issue of trade-offs in the evaluation of therapeutic technology.

SURROGATE VERSUS CLINICAL ENDPOINTS

The surrogate-versus-clinical endpoints battle is particularly prominent now in the drug arena. The issue is when new drugs should be released for clinical use. Under most circumstances, the Food and Drug Administration (FDA) has required evidence of clinical improvement and has rejected surrogate endpoints in making such decisions. The resultant delay has brought continuing opprobrium on the FDA. In a highly controversial and well-publicized decision, the FDA initially withheld approval of tissue-type plasminogen activator (t-PA), although evidence had been presented that t-PA lysed coronary thrombi and that arterial patency was achieved more frequently with t-PA than with streptokinase. But there was no evidence at the time that t-PA increased survival over that obtainable with streptokinase. Among the outraged critics of the decision was the Wall Street Journal which, under the headline "Human Sacrifice," mounted one of its many attacks on the regulatory bureaucracy of the FDA.

The FDA later did approve t-PA, which for a brief period appeared the treat-

16

ment of choice. Now there are beginning to be second thoughts. A New England Journal of Medicine report from New Zealand (1), showing no difference in ventricular function, coronary artery patency rates, and reinfarction—again, incidentally, surrogate endpoints—suggests that there is no difference between these two drugs other than cost. One should bear in mind that the sample size was small, with 130 and 135 patients receiving streptokinase and t-PA respectively. Of course, one major advantage of surrogate endpoints is that smaller sample sizes may be adequate. Even with such a small sample, it is interesting to note that after 30 days there were 10 deaths in patients receiving streptokinase and 5 in patients receiving t-PA; after 9 months there were 12 and 8 deaths respectively. While the differences in mortality may appear suggestive, the p-values, 0.2 and 0.34 for the two time periods, did not reach the conventional level of statistical significance.

The other major surrogate-versus-clinical endpoints battle has been fought over cancer chemotherapy. Again, the FDA has been denounced by the Wall Street Journal for foot-dragging. The question under debate is whether we should expedite the introduction of drugs and under what circumstances. It has always seemed to me that for most drugs the public is better served by the relatively measured and cautious policy adopted by the FDA. My personal view reflects a concern for the risks, both known and unknown, of hastily introduced technology. I believe it was Harold Green, chair of the 1973 Artificial Heart Assessment Panel, who suggested that a delay in introducing a new therapy means only that the public has to live with the status quo, while the widespread use of inadequately tested treatments can possibly expose the public to substantial harm. The views of potential recipients of treatment may be quite different, depending on the severity of the condition. While most of medicine is concerned with conditions that are not life-threatening, it is entirely appropriate that we adopt different attitudes and policies for introducing drugs which treat life-threatening conditions as opposed to those for treating the large proportion of routine medicine.

However well or cautiously we evaluate drugs in Phases I, II, and III, a major shortcoming in how we introduce drugs in this country is in follow-up. Once a drug has been introduced, we have no systematic and comprehensive way to detect or control long-term risks and benefits. It has been observed that Great Britain is willing to introduce drugs at an earlier stage in their development because the British system of post-marketing surveillance (PMS) may be more effective than the United States post-marketing system; see for instance the contribution of Inman in this volume. It is a source of considerable chagrin that our country failed to act on the recommendations of the President's Commission on Post-Marketing Surveillance that would have established a reliable system of PMS a decade ago.

The problem of post-marketing surveillance is at least as great for medical devices and procedures as for drugs. Surgeons in particular do not have good data on long-term outcomes. Note, for example, the incredulity of urologists who learned from John Wennberg's research about the number of patients who die within a year after transurethral resection of the prostate (see Chapter 4).

CLINICAL ENDPOINTS

I will return to the question of how good a surrogate for clinical endpoints an intermediate endpoint may be, but first it will be useful to examine the clinical endpoint itself: How reliable are clinical endpoints? Are they adequate gold standards themselves? The debate over condition-specific versus all-cause mortality is particularly interesting and sobering. It is well recognized that all-cause mortality is a purer endpoint than disease-specific deaths, because all-cause mortality helps avoid such problems as bias in patient selection, missing data, and changes in classification over time.

Proponents of new therapies understandably would prefer to judge their results on the basis of the specific condition the treatment is intended to relieve. An investigator might well ask why death from a completely unrelated cause should count against the proposed therapy. But it is not always clear that the "unrelated" cause is really unrelated. The latest example to come to my attention is a report from Scotland, in the British Medical Journal, in which the authors report an observational study correlating blood cholesterol levels with cardiac deaths and other endpoints, cancer in particular (2). The investigators found the predicted association between cholesterol level and cardiac deaths, but the reduction in cardiac deaths associated with lower cholesterol was offset by an equal increase in cancer deaths.

You may be familar with the unpleasant fact that in three major lipid drug trials, the fall in cardiac mortality associated with lower blood cholesterol was offset by increased accidental deaths in the experimental groups, and total mortality was unchanged (3,4,5). Investigators still are trying to figure out whether this awkward relationship between lower cholesterol and accidental deaths is causal.

Offsetting mortalities can, of course, go the other way. In studying the possible condition-specific mortality risk of a therapy, it is equally important to examine the possibility that the therapy produces an offsetting fall in total mortality. For example, in the National Halothane Study, we were concerned that some patients receiving the anesthetic halothane would die of liver failure. We were also aware of the possibility that halothane, because of its superior clinical properties, might have offsetting decreases in mortality from other causes. As it turned out, there were but a handful of deaths from liver necrosis, and these were more than offset by a fall in all-cause mortality for patients receiving halothane.

From the foregoing considerations, I posit that the phenomenon of offsetting risks is important and perhaps not adequately appreciated. It is by no means limited to mortality. Mortality is what we tend to study, not only because it is important, but also because it is easier to measure than many other things we would like to know and that are also important. When a technology intended to improve quality of life has both benefits and risks, they are likely to be very difficult to compare. It is the old apples-versus-oranges problem, but even worse since there may be several baskets of different fruits to be balanced in the equation.

Improvement in quality of life is not only an important outcome of medical care; it is the only intended outcome of most of what we do in medicine. In commenting on the failure of cholesterol-lowering drugs to reduce total mortality, Fries, Green, and Levine point out that "the primary purpose of most health promotion activities . . . is to improve quality of life" and that, by implication, it may be unrealistic to expect or demand that length of life be extended (6). More important, they suggest, is the decreased morbidity and improved quality of life that accompany a decrease in risk factors and improved cardiovascular function.

There are any number of therapies, intended to improve quality of life, which have offsetting adverse effects. I will mention a few: thalidomide causing phocomelia, diethylstilbestrol (DES) causing vaginal cancer in the offspring of women receiving it, swine flu vaccine followed by Guillain-Barré syndrome. The latter is of particular interest because a very large clinical trial was not large enough to pick up the rare but extremely serious syndrome. The ever-present risk of side effects, many unknown, with everyday treatment is part of the price we must pay when therapy is effective. It is not quite so easy to accept the inevitable complications and ill effects of other therapies, such as the severe malabsorption problems that followed gastric bypass surgery, metabolic imbalances that could have been easily predicted.

Two common operations that are performed to improve quality of life may have an opposite effect. As Wennberg et al. remind us, prostatectomy is often followed by impotence and incontinence (7). Hysterectomy may be followed by depression and an increase in urinary tract infections. Recent data suggest, however, that the improvements in quality of life for many or most patients undergoing elective hysterectomy or prostatectomy may more than offset the potential ill effects of the procedures. To balance the quality-of-life benefits and risks of such procedures we must consider the values of the patient. These depend heavily on how individual patients perceive the benefits and risks of the procedures. Unfortunately, we do not yet know how to present the issue of risk to patients in a meaningful way; nor, I suspect, do those of us in the profession fully understand these risks. It is clear, however, that different patients have different values, and that patients' values may differ widely from those ascribed to them by their physicians (8).

There is another difficulty. A quality-of-life therapy may have as its goal a single condition-specific benefit that is easily measurable, but we don't have any single all-cause index to identify and measure possible offsetting negative effects. Indeed, we may not even know what side effects to look for when a therapy is introduced. An observational study before introduction may, however, give us some clues as to potential side effects to look for in long-term surveillance.

As Chapter 4 indicates, all outcomes that are relevant to a patient should be included in evaluative research: mortality and morbidity, complications, symptom reduction, and functional status improvement, as well as the standard physiologic and biochemical surrogates. For this purpose, Fries and Spitz, in a recently published book, have proposed a hierarchy of quality-of-life assessment indices for surveillance: death, disability, discomfort, drug side effects, and dollar costs (9), each of the latter four subdivided into relevant components (e.g., pain, fatigue, depression, anxiety).

While it is of course desirable to obtain a definitive evaluation of a new product or treatment as soon as possible, haste can create serious problems, as we saw with t-PA. Another example of the importance of timing is the use of injected chymopapain as an alternative treatment for the relief of ruptured intervertebral disks. In clinical trials it appeared safe and effective. But serious complications (transverse myelitis and anaphylactoid reactions) were reported shortly after the FDA released chymopapain for general use (10). A third interesting and sobering example is the recent report that, in randomized clinical trials comparing mastectomy with mastectomy plus radiation to the chest wall for breast cancer, there was a late increase in serious cardiac events, coronary artery disease, and unrelated malignancies in the group receiving radiation (11). With t-PA and chymopapain the adverse effects were detected very quickly. With DES and with radiation in the foregoing example, they occurred much later. It may even be necessary to wait years.

Radiation techniques for breast cancer have changed and presumably improved considerably, so that patients undergoing lumpectomy and radiation now may be spared these complications, but we simply do not know if that is so. As Chapter 12 points out, devices and procedures are generally subject to incremental innovation. Not only will an operation or procedure differ among different physicians, but the procedure or device itself will be modified over time. It may be difficult ever to know when to evaluate devices and procedures and we may therefore need to follow patients for long periods. We need to invoke the right and accept the responsibility to review the effects of treatment continually, and to revise our clinical decisions as new evidence becomes available.

SURROGATE ENDPOINTS

Returning to surrogate endpoints: they have all the problems of clinical endpoints plus a good many of their own. They can be related only to condition-specific outcomes, and their relationship to hoped-for clinical outcomes may not be a strong one. I might point out that this is analogous to the well-known problem central to the medical audit, the process-versus-outcome relationship that we have all worried about.

The potential usefulness of surrogate endpoints during the early stages of development appears to be strongest in the cardiac area, but we have already seen the problems experienced with t-PA. The use of surrogate endpoints has also been explored with some enthusiasm for cancer chemotherapy, with shrinkage of tumor size the usual proposed surrogate for increased life expectancy. However strong the association between such surrogates and their intended effects may prove to be, a serious limitation of surrogates as a basis for evaluation is that none of the offsetting adverse effects can be determined when surrogate outcomes are used.

I would like to call your attention to the April 1989 issue of Statistics in Medicine, the first four articles of which are devoted to discussion of surrogate endpoints. They explore in depth three conditions that one might consider as having the greatest potential: cancer (12), cardiovascular disease (13), and ophthalmologic disorders (14). One advantage that is emphasized is that surrogates provide earlier answers. But it is of interest that, in its attempt to expedite the availability of drugs to treat AIDS and cancer, the FDA has not moved to allow surrogate endpoints; the enhanced speed is achieved by collapsing Phases II and III and giving such drugs priority treatment (J. Goyan, personal communication, 1989).

In conclusion, I will make four points. First, when dealing with mortality as an endpoint of treatment, all-cause mortality is ignored at the peril of the investigators and the public. Second, when dealing with quality of life, multiple or hierarchical endpoints must be considered; their identity may not be known in advance; and they cannot be summarized in a single number, for there is no all-cause quality of life equivalent of all-cause mortality. Third, a more systematic and comprehensive method of long-term monitoring or surveillance is needed. If one is established, a greater reliance on surrogate endpoints might be justified. Finally, we must be concerned with the complex issue of an informed public's wants and values.

REFERENCES

1. White HD, Rivers JT, Maslowski AH, et al. Effect of intravenous streptokinase as compared with that of tissue plasminogen activator on left ventricular function after first myocardial infarction. New England Journal of Medicine 1989;320:817–821.
2. Isles CG, Hole DJ, Gillis CR, Hawthorne VM, Lever AF. Plasma cholesterol, coronary heart disease, and cancer in Renfrew and Paisley survey. British Medical Journal 1989;298:920–924.
3. Frick MH, Elo O, Haapa K, Heinonen OP. Helsinki Heart Study: Primary-prevention trial with gemfibrozil in middle-aged men with dyslipidemia. New England Journal of Medicine 1987;317:1237–1245.

4. Coronary heart disease death, nonfatal acute myocardial infarction and other clinical outcomes in the Multiple Risk Factor Intervention Trial Research Group. American Journal of Cardiology 1986;58:1–13.

5. The Lipid Research Clinics Coronary Primary Prevention Trial results. I. Reduction of incidence of coronary heart disease. Journal of the American Medical Association 1984;251:351–364.

6. Fries JF, Green LW, Levine S. Health promotion and the compression of morbidity. Lancet 1989;1:481–483.

7. Wennberg JE, Roos N, Sola L, Schori A, Jaffe R. Use of claims data systems to evaluate health care outcomes: Morbidity and reoperation following prostatectomy. Journal of the American Medical Association 1987;257:933–936.

8. McNeil BJ, Weichselbaum R, Pauker SG. Fallacy of the five-year survival in lung cancer. New England Journal of Medicine 1978;299:1397.

9. Fries JF, Spitz PW. The hierarchy of patient outcomes. In Spilker B (ed.) Quality of Life Assessments in Clinical Trials. New York: Raven Press, 1990:25–35.

10. Blue Shield of California, Medical Policy Committee (March 4, 1987).

11. Houghton J, Baum M. Adjuvant radiotherapy in breast cancer: Considerations of cost-benefits in relation to the CRC (King's/Cambridge) trial. International Journal of Technology Assessment in Health Care 1989;5:415–422.

12. Ellenberg SS, Hamilton JM. Surrogate endpoints in clinical trials: Cancer. Statistics in Medicine 1989;8:405–413.

13. Wittes J, Latos E. Surrogate endpoints in clinical trials: Cardiovascular diseases. Statistics in Medicine 1989;8:415–426.

14. Hillis A, Seigel D. Surrogate endpoints in clinical trials: Ophthalmologic disorders. Statistics in Medicine 1989;8:427–430.

3

Advances in Health Status Measurement: The Potential to Improve Experimental and Non-Experimental Data Collection

MARILYN BERGNER

Advances in health status measurement have given us a choice of reliable and valid measures to use in clinical trials of drugs and devices. To use them, however, investigators may have to revise the design of trials and their data collection methods. The primary objective of this paper is to familiarize the reader with current health status measures. The secondary objectives are almost equally important. They are to examine the way clinical trials are conducted, to distinguish between quality of life and health status measures, to suggest modifications necessary to incorporate health status measures into clinical trials, and to discuss four problems that are often cited as barriers to the use of health status measures.

THE CONDUCT OF CLINICAL TRIALS

Phase II or Phase III clinical trials of new drugs and medical devices are generally conducted in the following fashion. They generally take place in many medical centers throughout the country and sometimes even in several countries. The incentive for the participation of these centers or of physicians is the fee received for patients enrolled in the trial. Usually the fee is meant to cover the cost of data collection, including personnel and additional testing. Each center hires staff or assigns existing staff to collect the needed information. Since the health professionals participating in the trial are those providing clinical care, they usually are principally expert in clinical medicine rather than evaluative research.

The design of trials and data collection forms is done by the coordinating center—usually a department of the firm running the study. The format of these

23

data collection instruments is often a compromise between completeness, ease of recording by the primary data collector, ease of conversion to computer-readable form, and ease of analysis. The ones I have seen tend to be closely packed with questions, with limited space for answers. Some questions are straightforward: What is the patient's blood pressure? But some of them require judgment: What size is the mass? Is the tumor shrinking? Has the patient had any side effects? There are few or no guidelines about the kind of information that must be provided to answer these questions.

The data collected in these trials refer only to the patients enrolled in the study. No information is obtained about patients who were considered for enrollment but, for one reason or another, were not approached by the physician or staff members. Furthermore, patients often drop out without anyone inquiring why they left. The dropout is sometimes recorded on the chart or form but, more often than not, the only source of that information is the physician.

Finally, these studies generally are designed, implemented, and supervised by statisticians whose expertise is in analytic design and data analysis. Their training and experience usually do not prepare them to guard against errors related to biases in enrollment or unreliability of data. No matter how sophisticated the design of a study and no matter how skilled the analysis, unreliable data and selective enrollment of patients can undermine even a randomized trial.

Trials designed in this fashion leave little or no room for the collection of data about health status. However, some studies do include health status measures. How have these studies been designed and conducted? Answering this question requires one to recognize that health status is not the term ordinarily used when clinical investigators want to examine treatment effects that are not biomedical. Instead, quality of life is assessed. Now, is there a difference between health status and quality of life?

MEASUREMENT OF QUALITY OF LIFE AND OF HEALTH STATUS

Quality of life is not defined in the reports of clinical trials that I have read. The reader must deduce a definition from the dimensions[1] that are assessed. A review of the literature shows that quality of life may include any one or a combination of the following factors: physical activity, social and leisure activity, work, symptoms, loss of income, cognition, emotional adaptation, self-esteem,

---

[1]The word dimension refers to an area of interest or concern that is measured by several interrelated variables. For example, cardiovascular function is a dimension of health measured by blood pressure, treadmill performance, EKG, etc.; mental status is a dimension of health that may be measured by cognitive level, mood, effect, etc.

TABLE 3.1 Suggested domains of quality of life

Symptoms	Emotional status
Functional status	Anxiety
Self care	Stress
Mobility	Depression
Physical activity	Locus of control
Role activities	Spiritual well-being
Work	Cognition
Household management	Sleep and rest
Social functioning	Energy and vitality
Personal interactions	Health perceptions
Intimacy	General life satisfaction
Community interactions	

anxiety, stress, sexual activity, interpersonal relationships, impotence, incontinence, and overall satisfaction with life. Each investigation that purports to address quality of life actually examines a very narrow set of factors. Reasons for the choice of factors are rarely made clear, nor are the reasons for omitting elements that might be relevant.

Table 3.1 provides a list of dimensions of quality of life that were suggested by conferees at a workshop on quality of life and cardiovascular disease. You should note the breadth of the dimensions covered and the fact that there is no suggestion of the interrelationship between dimensions.

Conceptual frameworks for health status, on the other hand, have appeared in the literature, have been extensively discussed, and have provided the underpinnings of several measures. One of these conceptualizations is given in Table 3.2. This table indicates the dimensions that constitute health status and how they relate to one another. It is clearly concerned with health, not with other aspects of life which may influence its quality.

Systematic measures of functional status have been used by clinical researchers for more than 50 years. The first were developed to assess the baseline performance status of participants in clinical research projects. In some cases they were used to determine patient eligibility for participation in a trial. The Karnofsky Performance Status Index, the New York Heart Association Classification, and the Specific Activity Scale are examples. They have at least three distinguishing characteristics: they are brief, with patients assigned to one of no more than ten categories; each is specific to a particular disease or condition; and they usually are completed by a physician on the basis of observation and history of the patient.

All these measures of functional status were developed by physicians or other clinicians to systematize the collection and recording of information thought relevant for diagnosis and treatment; none was subjected to rigorous

TABLE 3.2 The dimensions of health status

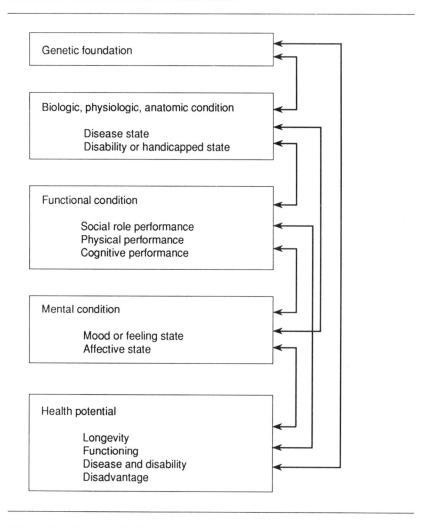

Adapted from Bergner, M. Measurement of Health Status. Medical Care 1985;23:696

development and testing. Thus, their reliability tends to be poor, which precludes their use for monitoring patient progress or assessing outcome of therapy. This does not mean that they are not used for these purposes. In fact, they are probably the most commonly used measures of quality of life. However, none of them requires that the patients be asked directly about the characteristics assessed, even though the recorder—a doctor or nurse—may not have the information necessary to provide a reliable assessment.

In sharp contrast with these measures is a group of measures, called health status measures, which have been developed relatively recently and have a general focus. All of them include physical functioning, but they also include other aspects of health; these may be symptoms, emotional status, cognition, or perceptions of health.

The developers of health status measures expected their results to be valuable for formulating health policy, since they provide information about the health status of populations and about the benefits of new therapies or systems of health services delivery, such as increased use of home health services. These purposes are distinct from those articulated by the developers of measures for use in clinical practice.

Because the group of measures aimed at clinical research was not intended for routine use in a physician's office, however, developers were not concerned with the amount of time it would add to a patient visit, whether the doctor, patient, nurse, or receptionist would complete it, or whether the number of questions was small enough to be tolerated by the staff. In fact, in most cases the aims were directly opposite to those encountered in developing a measure of health status for clinical practice. They were:

- the need to be comprehensive, so that all aspects of health status were included;
- the need to specify a method for answering the questions that did not involve clinicians; and
- the need to assure reliable measurement (which often means longer measures) because the research setting precludes assurance that a nurse or physician will determine the reliability of a response.

Many of these general health status measures have been carefully developed and are used extensively. They provide hard data that are reliable and reproducible. In fact, the data they produce are often more reliable than physiologic data. What physiologic test has a reliability coefficient of .90? Several health status measures do. A valuable discussion of the various general measures is provided in Measuring Health, by McDowell and Newell (1). Table 3.3, taken from this book, lists some general health status measures.

In addition to these general health status measures, disease-specific measures have been used in clinical research. The rationale for their development and use is that they address the specific concerns of the clinical entity being investigated, they can be shorter than the general measures, and they may be more sensitive to the changes that occur with treatment. All the new disease-specific measures have been developed with the same care as the general measures. They do not ask for a clinician's judgment about the patient's condition, and they meet stringent reliability standards.

TABLE 3.3 Comparison of the quality of general health measurements

Measurement	Scale	Number of items	Application	Administered by (time)	Studies using method	Reliability Testing thoroughness	Reliability Results	Validity Testing thoroughness	Validity Results
Arthritis Impact Measurement Scale AIMS) (Meenan)	ordinal (Guttman)	45	clinical	self (15 min.)	few	++	++	++	++
Physical and Mental Impairment-of-Function Evaluation (PAMIE) (Gurel)	ordinal	77	clinical	expert (10-15 min.)	few	+	++	+	+
Functional Assessment Inventory (Crewe and Athelstan)	ordinal	40	clinical	expert (5 min.)	few	++	++	++	++
Nottingham Health Profile (Martini and Hunt)	interval	38	clinical, survey	self (<10 min.)	several	++	++	++	++
Sickness Impact Profile (Bergner)	interval	136	survey	self (20-30 min.)	many	++	+++	++	++
Multilevel Assessment Instrument (Lawton)	ordinal	147	survey	interviewer (50 min.)	few	++	++	++	++
Multidimensional Functional Assessment Questionnaire (OARS)	ordinal	120	clinical (Part A)	interviewer (30 min.)	several	++	++	++	++
CORE-CARE (Gurland)	ordinal	329	clinical	interviewer	several	++	++	++ (full CARE, not CORE-CARE)	++
Quality of Well-Being Scale (Bush)	ratio	18	research	interviewer (15 min.)	several	++	+++	+	++

SOURCE: McDowell I, Newell C. Measuring Health: A Guide to Rating Scales and Questionnaires. New York: Oxford University Press. 1987:270.

INCLUSION OF QUALITY OF LIFE AND HEALTH STATUS
MEASURES IN CLINICAL TRIALS

Despite the availability of health status measures, quality of life measurement in clinical trials is often an afterthought. Clinical trials are designed to examine a medical outcome: tumor shrinkage, longevity, pulmonary function, renal function, level of angina, shortness of breath, and so on. But what happens when, long after all aspects of the research have been settled, someone realizes that the therapy may affect aspects of a person's life that are not strictly medical. It may not be pleasant to become bald and nauseated, to eat a restricted diet, or to be tied to a machine for 12 of 24 hours. Because such consequences of treatment and treatment-related side effects can affect all aspects of a patient's life, a quality of life assessment is deemed necessary.

This assessment must meet certain criteria, however: it must fit into the planned data collection scheme; it must be short so as not to burden the patient; it must take no more than 15 minutes of the data collector's time; and it must be immediately acceptable and understandable to all the clinical members of the research team. These are formidable requirements which often preclude the use of well-developed health status measures. Furthermore, while the collection of biomedical data for clinical trials may require the skills of a clinician, health status data are particularly prone to biases that can be introduced by clinicians. The most obvious bias is the possibility that patients will not provide accurate information if they believe it will embarrass the clinician or reflect poorly on their own behavior.

Nonetheless, drug companies and manufacturers of medical devices have become consumers of quality of life and health status assessments. At one time their interest in this area was confined to very specific side effects. That has changed over the past few years, for two reasons. One is the demand of third-party payers for more extensive evidence of the benefits of new drugs and devices, especially when they may be more costly. The other is the marketing advantage that may accrue if a new drug is shown to improve quality of life.

Drug companies have undertaken a large number of quality of life and health status studies. Unfortunately, most of them are not published. In fact, only two have been, the captopril and auranofin trials (2,3), and I, for one, am tired of hearing about them as the harbingers of good things to come. What is interesting about these two studies, however, is their differences. The auranofin trial used well-developed multidimensional general measures that provide a health status score for each patient. The captopril study used a hodgepodge of independent measures to assess a variety of factors including distress, fatigue, impotence, and cognition. Some measures had already been developed, some were modifications of existing measures, and some were newly developed for the study. There was no way to combine the measures into a single index score. Most distressing to those of us in the field, the measures themselves are not available to other investigators. Though I am aware of several other drug and device studies that have used health status measures, they have not been published and information about them is difficult if not impossible to obtain.

I also know of studies that were never implemented or were sharply curtailed because manufacturers feared they would provide unfavorable evidence about products. After all, if the patient is asked about a series of symptoms or problems or dysfunctions that may be interpreted as side effects, some may turn up. If, on the other hand, only the physician provides this information, it is usually filtered by selective questioning of the patient. Thus, no unexpected or unlikely effects—good or bad—generally are found.

Aquired immune deficiency syndrome (AIDS) provides a perfect example of this. There was early evidence that AZT might have some deleterious side effects, but there was little interest in systematic examination of these effects. Only now that some work has been done by independent investigators does there seem to be interest by those directly involved in the development of new AIDS drugs in examining these effects.

FOUR PROBLEMS REGARDING THE MEASUREMENT OF HEALTH STATUS IN CLINICAL TRIALS

My review of clinical research that assesses health status identified four broad issues: conceptualization of a construct, the value of a gold standard, the clinical significance and sensitivity of the measures, and practical administrative problems.

The major issue is conceptualization. The terms quality of life, health status, and functional status are often used interchangeably and without definition. Clinical investigators naively ask about a measure of quality of life, as if there were a single best exemplar to be used in all cases. Quality of life, like health or illness, must be assessed specifically. Although a few basic measurements (such as temperature; blood pressure; difficulty eating, sleeping, or dressing) may apply to everyone in every situation, many more are relevant only to particular patients (such as glomerular filtration, ejection fraction, pain, impotence, walking, cognition). Each investigator must think about a study in terms of the intervention and patients involved, and decide what to assess. In general, the assessment should examine factors that are likely to be affected by the intervention, factors that may be affected, and factors that are unlikely to occur but are possible. Once the dimensions or categories are identified, appropriate measures can be selected for use.

Somewhere in the process of deciding on dimensions and choosing measures, clinical investigators often start a futile search for the gold standard that everyone will find appropriate and credible. The bitter truth is that there is no gold standard, there is unlikely ever to be one, and it is unlikely that one is desirable. Health, like intelligence, is a complex attribute that requires a multidimensional measure. There is no gold standard for intelligence tests. Many are psychometrically sound and have been used enough to assure investigators

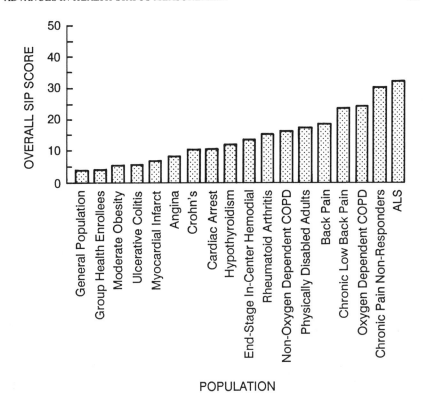

POPULATION

FIGURE 3.1 Overall Sickness Impact Profile (SIP) scores for different disease conditions or population groups. SOURCE: Patrick DL, Deyo RA. Generic and disease-specific measures in assessing health status and quality of life. In: Advances in Health Status Assessment: Conference Proceedings. Medical Care 1989;27(3):S220.

that they "work." The choice of a test depends on the particular situation. However, intelligence tests do have an important advantage over measures of health status. They have been used enough that the meaning of a score is understood, and a difference of three or five or ten points can be translated, however crudely, into a mental picture of what the person can do. When individuals differ, there is confidence that the test will pick up the difference.

The clinical importance of score differences and health status is still unclear, and the meaning of any particular score on a health status measure produces no mental pictures that represents real people or real patients. However, a recently published article may soon remedy this situation a bit (4). Patrick and Deyo have reviewed many studies that used the Sickness Impact Profile, one of the more commonly applied general health status measures, and put together Figure 3.1.

The administrative problems that I have alluded to are not easily solved. They are principally concerned with determination of health status for those persons for whom current measures may be inappropriate. These include the emotionally or cognitively impaired, the illiterate, those not proficient in English, and those not familiar with American culture. These problems are inherent in obtaining any data that require communication with a patient, not only health status measures.

The advantage of health status measures is that we know how they should behave if they are used properly. If investigators use measures that are well developed, they may become convinced that they need not develop something new for each trial. That step alone would increase the efficiency of clinical trials. It would also begin to develop a body of experience that could advance the acceptance of such measures by regulatory agencies. With such acceptance may come a greater appreciation of the importance of health-related quality of life as a major goal of technology development.

REFERENCES

1. McDowell I, Newell C. Measuring Health: A Guide to Rating Scales and Questionnaires. New York: Oxford University Press, 1987:270.
2. Croog SH, Levine S, Testa MA, Brown B, Bulpitt CJ, Jenkins CD, Klerman GL, Williams GH. The effects of antihypertensive therapy on the quality of life. New England Journal of Medicine 1986;314:1657–1664.
3. Bombardier C, Ware J, Russell IJ, Larson M, Chalmers A, Read JL. Auranofin therapy and quality of life in patients with rheumatoid arthritis: Results of a multicenter trial. American Journal of Medicine 1986;81:565–578.
4. Patrick DL, Deyo, RA. Generic and disease-specific measures in assessing health status and quality of life. In: Lohr KN (ed.) Advances in Health Status Assessment: Conference Proceedings. 1989;27:S217–S232.

4

What Is Outcomes Research?

JOHN E. WENNBERG

In "The Structure of Scientific Revolutions" Thomas Kuhn suggests that science is what scientists do. I want to take my cue from him and will discuss what our research team is doing that we call outcomes research. I then will return to Kuhn to make some more general observations about the status of outcomes research and the emergence of evaluative clinical sciences as a response to medicine's current predicament.

WHICH RATE IS RIGHT?

For some time, our research group has been conducting a series of investigations of the outcomes of treatment for benign prostatic hyperplasia (BPH). These investigations are part of an effort to come to terms with the puzzling geographic variations in rates of use of medical care. By the mid 1970s, I had become convinced that these variations exist primarily because of differences in physician practice style, and that a resolution of the puzzle required direct inquiry into the effect on outcome of the various opinions or clinical theories underlying these practice styles (1). By the early 1980s, Dan Hanley, David Soule, and Alice Russell had organized leading physicians in Maine into study groups to investigate the variations (2). These study groups became the focus of an alliance between practicing physicians and researchers that made many of our studies possible.

Of these studies, the assessments of alternative treatments for BPH have become the most widely known, and it is fair to say that it is in the groping for solutions to the problems associated with BPH that our understanding of outcomes research has developed the furthest (3-7). The BPH study group, organized in 1982 by Robert Timothy, consists largely of practicing urologists. Our BPH assessment team consists of research urologists, medical care epidemiologists, decision analysts, statisticians, psychometricians, computer scientists, and experts in interactive videodisc technology (see Table 4.1).

At issue is the treatment of prostatism or obstruction of the urinary tract due to benign hyperplasia of the prostate gland. BPH is a very common condition, affecting the majority of men by the seventh or eighth decade of life. One com-

TABLE 4.1 Members of the BPH Assessment Team

Discipline	Members	Location
Biostatistics	Klim McPherson	Oxford, U.K.
Clinical Decision Analysis	Michael J. Barry	Boston, MA
	Albert G. Mulley	Boston, MA
Computer Science/Interactive Videodisc Technology	Eric Baumgartner	Hanover, NH
	J. Robert Beck	Hanover, NH
	Joseph V. Henderson	Washington, DC
	Harold C. Lyon, Jr.	Hanover, NH
	Barbara Sasso	Hanover, NH
	Coralea Wennberg	Hanover, NH
Medical Care Epidemiology/ Claims Data Studies	Nicolas Black	London, U.K.
	Thomas A. Bubolz	Hanover, NH
	Marsha M. Cohen	Manitoba, Canada
	Elliott S. Fisher	Hanover, NH
	E. Robert Greenberg	Hanover, NH
	David J. Malenka	Hanover, NH
	Dale McLerran	Hanover, NH
	Aviva Ron	Tel Aviv, Israel
	Leslie L. Roos	Manitoba, Canada
	Noralou P. Roos	Manitoba, Canada
	John H. Wasson	Hanover, NH
	John E. Wennberg	Hanover, NH
Medical Ethics	Charles Culver	Hanover, NH
Psychometrics/ Survey Research	Tavs Folmer Anderson	Copenhagen, Denmark
	Floyd J. Fowler	Boston, MA
Urology	Reginald Bruskewitz	Madison, WI
	Abraham Cockett	Rochester, NY
	John A. Heaney	Hanover, NH
	H. Logan Holtgrewe	Annapolis, MD
	Ernest Ramsey	Manitoba, Canada
	Stuart M. Selikowitz	White River Jct., VT
	Robert P. Timothy	Portland, ME

mon treatment for BPH is an operation, a prostatectomy. The rate of prostatectomy varies strikingly among neighboring communities. In some places about
10 percent of men undergo this operation by age 85, while in other communities
the proportion can be as high as 50 percent. In 1987, some 340,000 prostatectomies were performed for BPH at a cost of roughly $4 billion. Another com-
mon treatment for BPH is watchful waiting. In communities with low rates of
prostatectomy, proportionately more men with BPH are treated by this alternative strategy. Clinical practice in these communities emphasizes the viewpoint
that prostatectomy is an elective procedure, reserved for those with truly bur-
densome symptoms.

The assessment of BPH started with a discussion between the researchers
and the members of the study group, who represented many geographic areas in
Maine with considerable variations in rates of surgery. This discussion focused
on establishing the different points of view or clinical theories behind these geographic variations. Together with a review of the scientific papers published on
BPH, it uncovered an important and unsettled controversy concerning the indications for the operation. Many physicians hold the theory that prostatectomy
should be performed early in the course of BPH as a preventive measure. They
reason that if the operation is delayed, the patient will be older and at higher
risk when it finally becomes unavoidable; if the operation is delayed, life
expectancy is reduced. According to this theory, watchful waiting is not a reasonable option for most patients. Other physicians argue that the need for the
operation is not inevitable, that it does not improve life expectancy for most
patients and that the primary reason for surgery is relief of symptoms and
improvement in the quality of life. According to this theory, watchful waiting is
a reasonable option for patients who prefer to live with their symptoms to avoid
the risks of surgery (4-6).

The assessment team tested this conflict in theory and reached several conclusions. Evidence from the literature and from claims data demonstrated that
the preventive theory was incorrect: an operation in patients with uncomplicat-
ed BPH—which most patients have—very likely causes a slight decrease in life
expectancy. The assessment thus confirmed the opinion of those physicians
who felt the operation was justified because it reduces symptoms and improves
the quality of life. Interview studies with patients before surgery and at three,
six, and twelve months after surgery documented changes in symptom and functional status related to the operation. These studies showed that the value of the
operation for most patients is that it is better than watchful waiting for reducing
symptoms and improving quality of life. However, these gains are available
only to patients willing to take the risks of the operation, which include death,
failure to improve symptoms, impotence, and incontinence. The decision to
undergo the operation is thus highly dependent on patients' preferences for outcomes and their attitudes toward risk.

This substantial clarification of theory occurred without a prospective clinical trial; the steps undertaken and the disciplines involved are listed in Table 4.2. Note the emphasis on study groups with physicians to learn about their theories of treatment, and focus groups with patients to learn about the expectations and outcomes that matter to them. The literature review and the claims data provided enough information to define the actuarial expectations for the operated and unoperated patient (without chronic retention) and to test the preventive theory of early prostatectomy. We had to depend on the placebo arm of a few drug trials and a scant series of four studies of BPH patients treated with watchful waiting for estimates of the natural history of symptoms and the frequency of crossover to operation. We found no satisfactory information on symptom relief after surgery in the literature, so we conducted our own study. The results provide convincing evidence that the operation is much more effective than watchful waiting as a treatment for BPH symptoms. Thus, there is no dispute about the "main effect" superiority of surgery over watchful waiting. Decision analysis, used to test the preventive theory, also demonstrates that the decision to undergo the operation depends on patient attitudes toward impotence, incontinence, and the operative mortality rate. The subjective factors of risk aversion and personal tolerance for disease symptoms thus emerge as important elements of rational choice.

The BPH assessment had immediate practical value for clinical decision making because it clarified controversies, established correct theory, and providing detailed probability estimates, some of which had not been previously studied. The effect of practice style on variation in prostatectomy rates was traced to an incorrect belief in the preventive theory of early prostatectomy and

TABLE 4.2 Synopsis of BPH assessment: Prostatectomy versus watchful waiting

Steps Used in the BPH Assessment	Evaluative Clinical Sciences: Methods/Disciplines
Identify treatment theories and evaluate	Structured review of the literature; meta-analysis; focus groups with physicians
Identify and develop measures of relevant outcomes from patient's and from physician's points of view	Study focus groups; algorithms using claims data; patient interview instruments
Undertake non-experimental studies to estimate (missing) outcomes probabilities	Claims data studies; interview studies of surgery patients
Integrate information from all sources to test preventive theory and evaluate importance of patient utilities	Decision analysis used as "thought experiment"

failure to take patient preferences into account when recommending prostatecto-my. The remedy for unwanted practice-style variations, we concluded, requires the active engagement of the patient in the decision. It requires informing physicians and patients of the risks and benefits of prostatectomy and its alter-native, watchful waiting.

ENGAGING PATIENTS IN THE DECISION PROCESS

We are seeking new ways to engage patients in the decision process and to make our detailed probability estimates available to patients and physicians in "real time" for use in clinical decision making. To do this, we have developed a "BPH Shared Medical Decision Making Procedure" based on interactive videodisc technology. This interactive program can be used in the physician's office after standardized information on health status and physical condition is entered into the data base. The patient is asked to provide information about symptoms, functional status, and the strength of his feelings about them. This information allows us to identify the relevant prognostic subgroup to which the patient belongs so that a patient can be given the best available estimate.

The patient is then shown an audiovisual narration depicting the available choices, their possible outcomes, and associated probabilities. Interviews with two physician-patients (one who chose watchful waiting and the other prostatec-tomy) convey to the patient that there is indeed a choice; if physicians choose differently, so can their patients. Other interviews are testimonies about the principal outcomes, including an example of a complication associated with either choice. The interactive computer feature of the Shared Medical Decision Making Procedure means that information on the probabilities for outcomes is specific to the patient's subgroup, according to symptom severity and age. The patient can also exercise options to learn more about issues of particular con-cern and can review the presentation. At the end, the patient is given a printed synopsis to discuss with family and physician. The physician then helps the patient make a decision.

The BPH assessment conducted so far does clarify controversies in basic clinical theory and provides better estimates than previously available for symp-tom status. But important uncertainties remain about some probabilities that are important for patients with BPH who are trying to evaluate risk. The attributable postoperative (30-day) risk of death for prostatectomy remains unclear. For patients who underwent surgery, the sample on which estimates of symptom improvement and incontinence are based is small (about 400), so the standard deviations are sometimes large. For untreated patients, the situation is even less satisfactory. Given a watchful waiting situation, we were unable to obtain an accurate estimate of the chance of a second episode of acute retention. This information is important for helping patients who present with acute reten-tion to decide on treatment. The characteristics of the watchful waiting subgroup at risk for progression to chronic obstruction (with the potential for bladder decompensation) are also unclear.

The interactive videodisc program can help fill in these missing probability estimates because it is also a tool for outcomes research. At the first viewing, the patient can be enrolled in a prospective study of outcomes based on his choice of treatment—a cohort study that we call a preference trial. For outcomes research, the patient must return later (e.g., after 3, 6, or 24 months), regardless of type of treatment, at which point additional information about health and satisfaction with choice is entered into the data base. These data, accumulated over time and for many patients, can be used by researchers to update the information presented to future patients. In this way, the device participates in its own update and helps improve the scientific basis of medicine. We also plan research protocols to improve our understanding of the "framing" effects of our data displays and to learn more about helping patients make decisions consistent with their preferences. An important objective of these research protocols is to learn more about, and improve the role of, the physician as counselor and "cognitive" advisor to patients.

EXTENDING ASSESSMENT TO ALL RELEVANT TREATMENT THEORIES

In the course of our work we have encountered a number of other theories or controversies concerning the treatment of BPH. One is an "old" theory that the transurethral approach to prostatectomy has better outcomes than the open prostatectomy. Another is that prazosin and other alpha-blockage drugs used to treat hypertension are useful treatments for symptoms of BPH. We also found new techniques for treating BPH based on balloon dilation and identified two promising drugs undergoing FDA evaluation, a less invasive operative technique (prostatotomy), and a microwave diathermy treatment which is thought to relieve symptoms by reducing prostate size through the scarring of tissue. As our thinking about our role has evolved, we have come to see the advantages of having the assessment team include all alternative treatments, the old as well as the emerging. We therefore want to address the evaluative challenges each of these theories presents.

With the exception of the relative effectiveness of transurethral prostatectomy (TURP) versus open prostatectomy (an issue I will address below), these theories are quite new and few data exist on which to base an evaluation. The need for prospective evaluation thus arises. There is a debate within our group concerning approaches to prospective evaluation. We began with the orthodox view that a double-blind, placebo-controlled randomized clinical trial (RCT) is the optimal strategy for establishing the probability for outcomes of alternative treatments, but some of us are no longer sure that this is always the case. Our debate is not about the recognized difficulties of RCTs, such as the issue of placebo controls and patient blinding when surgery is involved, the problems of costs, logistics, and changing technology that can befuddle studies where end-points require many years of follow-up, or the problem posed by rare diseases where cases are few and far between. Our conclusions about the importance of patient preferences for rational decision making, at least in the treatment of BPH, raise questions about the role of randomization itself.

The first question concerns the ethical requirements for shared decision making and the legal requirements for informed consent. When the outcomes of alternative treatments for a given condition are asymmetric in some significant dimension—say, known differences in the risk of death—patient preferences with regard to what is known about these risks should influence treatment assignments. This is a strong challenge for the planning of further studies of watchful waiting versus TURP, where the uncertainty is not even about the "main treatment effect" probabilities, but about prognosis in certain subgroups on the watchful waiting arm. When informed about this uncertainty, few patients who want to share responsibility for decision making are indifferent to randomization. In this case, the most efficient and ethical way to obtain the missing probabilities and characterize patient subgroups may well be a preference trial—the systematic follow-up of patient cohorts where treatment assignments are made according to informed patient choice rather than by randomization.

A similar problem may exist in the evaluation of drugs such as prazosin. In this situation, the "main effect" probabilities concerning symptom relief are unknown and the rationale for randomization seems more compelling. However, Phase I safety studies (and the vast experience gained with prazosin in its use as an antihypertensive drug) show that mortality, over the short term at least, is lower than that following surgery, and that the drug does not cause incontinence. Again, when informed, few patients who want to share responsibility for decision making accept randomization.

The unwillingness of informed patients to accept randomization may not be the main point, however. The more important issue may be which approach provides the more useful information. To understand this, we need to know a good deal more about the confounding effects of study design on probability estimates, particularly for soft outcomes. A pragmatic view is that the information generated by clinical trials is useful only to the extent that it helps decide choice of treatment. When choice is delegated to the physician, the physician alone makes the connection between the evidence from clinical trials and the patient. In this case, the probabilities obtained under randomized designs that ignored or minimized the importance of patient preferences may be the best estimates for decisions. Under the shared decision making paradigm, however, it is not self-evident that classic RCTs provide the most accurate information.

Imagine a clinical trial of prazosin in which patients with BPH are randomly assigned to a preference trial or an RCT. Patient characteristics (co-morbidities, symptom status, demographics, etc.) are obtained before patients are given information about their choice. A modified version of the Shared Medical Decision Making Procedure (described above) is needed to present information uniformly to patients in all cooperating centers. On one arm of the trial, patients are offered surgery, watchful waiting, or the opportunity to participate in a double-blind, placebo-controlled randomized clinical trial of prazosin, based on the full disclosure of information which the ethics of shared patient decision making requires. On the other arm, they are offered a preference trial—the opportunity to elect surgery, watchful waiting, or prazosin, based on the same disclosure about what is known (and not known) about the effect of the drug. Patients who want additional information or advice before deciding on treatment are counseled by physicians operating under standard protocols who do not administer treatments. Follow-up to determine outcomes is by observers who are blinded as to treatment received. I have diagrammed such a trial in Figure 4.1.

The trial would explore a number of interesting problems. Would more patients elect the drug if they knew they would get it than would elect the double-blind trial? Would the subgroup of patients electing the double-blind trial fairly represent those who elect prazosin with the knowledge that they will get their choice of treatment? That is, would the probabilities for symptom reduction and other outcomes estimated in the double-blind trial be the same as those estimated in the preference trial? It seems to me they would not. Patients who agree to randomization after a fair presentation of the treatment dilemmas are very likely different from those who choose prazosin. Moreover, I suspect that the outcomes associated with freely chosen treatments will be more positive.

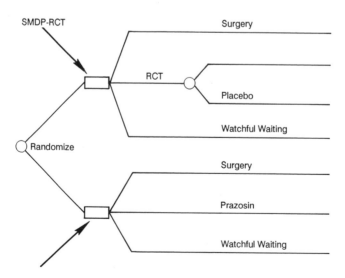

FIGURE 4.1 Proposed trial of a trial: Preference design versus double-blind randomized design.

The preference effect I am postulating is the common-sense notion that a treatment chosen by patients who believe it will help them is more likely to have a positive effect than randomly assigned treatments.

Studies of the effect of patient compliance in double-blinded RCTs provide some strong hints about the importance of the preference effect. David Sackett has found five documented instances where patients who comply with treatment regimens have substantially better outcomes, including survival, than noncompliant patients, even on the placebo arm of the trial. Which set of probabilities is most relevant to the everyday clinical situation? Under the shared decision making paradigm, the answer seems intuitively clear. The correct probabilities are those based on preference trials, where patients knowingly choose treatments on the basis of information about probabilities for the outcomes relevant to them. However, reliance on preference trials makes sense only if we can distinguish therapeutic effects from the effects of preference, placebo, and compliance. The trial I have proposed to you, because it also studies patients who choose watchful waiting and provides a complete accounting of choice and outcomes on both major arms of the study, may allow us to disentangle these effects.

Under the paradigm of shared decision making, what has been viewed as a distinct boundary between clinical research and everyday clinical practice promises to become blurred. The tools that help patients make informed choice also are useful for organizing clinical studies. The preference trial approach may prove more acceptable to practicing physicians and increase the possibility for large-scale, cooperative studies. It is somewhat of a scandal that, although prostatectomies have been performed since the beginning of this century and more than 350,000 are now performed annually in the United States, fewer than 400 patients—our series in Maine—have been followed systematically to study the "main effect" outcome, the effect of the operation on symptom status. The information on symptom status and crossover to operation for patients choosing watchful waiting is based on only four studies of a small series of non-operated patients.

I believe that many more patients will elect experimental treatments under preference designs than under randomized designs. If this is so, and if we become confident about the limitations and advantages of preference trials, this change will greatly speed the process and reduce the costs of technology assessment as well as provide new methods for Phase IV studies. For example, prazosin is now used extensively in everyday clinical practice in this country, but in order for its manufacturer to advocate its use for the treatment of BPH it must undergo an extensive series of RCTs. For all this trouble we would know little more than its relative value compared to a placebo; we would know nothing about the probabilities that count in clinical practice, such as its relative effectiveness compared to watchful waiting or surgery, and its value when patients freely choose their treatments. My hope is that our assessment team can broaden the investigation of the relative advantages of preference versus randomized clinical trials across the full spectrum of assessment issues we have encountered, including the merits of balloon dilation, microwave diathermy, and several new drugs.

We also need to consider the value of both trial designs in resolving another treatment controversy: the relative effectiveness of two surgical approaches to the prostate—the transurethral or the open prostatectomy. Over the past three decades, TURP has virtually replaced the older open operative techniques. This replacement, which occurred without prospective clinical trials, reflects the belief that TURP is a safer, less invasive operation that is effective in the long term. Since the administrative data bases available to our team extend back to the 1960s, we have compared the outcomes of these two operations over a considerable span of time. The results indicate that the open operation may be more effective. Patients with an open operation have significantly lower rates for stricture and reoperation, suggesting that the more complete removal of the prostate following the open operation, which is less traumatizing to the urethra, results in better long-term reduction of urinary symptoms. More puzzling and disturbing is the unexplained elevation in risk of death in the years following TURP. In separate studies undertaken in Maine (U.S.A.), Manitoba (Canada), Oxford (U.K.), and Denmark, we find the risk of death is significantly higher in the five years following operation.

In view of our concern that the higher mortality following TURP may occur because those patients are sicker than those undergoing open prostatectomy, we abstracted data on severity of illness from the medical charts at a large university hospital. Even after adjustment, however, the 45 percent higher mortality rate following TURP was unchanged. The consistency of the findings, and our failure to explain them on the basis of data available in medical charts, led us to conclude that differences in co-morbidity do not explain the effect and that a prospective study is needed to evaluate this problem.

Over the past several months, our assessment team has been in contact with urologists in various countries, including the leadership of the American Urological Association (AUA). We are extremely pleased that AUA has urged its members to participate in a large-scale clinical trial. The clinical trial being planned will not concentrate solely on the open versus TURP controversy. Since the available data suggest that TURP does harm, we have reasoned that this harm, if a true effect, will reveal itself no matter what the comparison group. The clinical trial thus provides the opportunity for direct comparison of new technologies—balloon dilation, microwave diathermy, and the new drugs—with surgery and watchful waiting. We hope that the clinical trial will provide the essential information on the outcome of all new treatment theories relevant to treatment of BPH.

We emphasize randomization in this situation for several reasons. It would be unwise to base the primary test of open prostatectomies versus TURP on a preference trial, because the necessary methodologic work to understand the limits and advantages of preference trials has not been done. The controversy here is about the role of patient risk factors as the confounding variables responsible for higher mortality rates following TURP. Well-conducted and large-scale randomized clinical trials give assurance that patient differences do not confound treatment effects. Moreover, it is ethical to randomize if the patient will accept randomization: our assessment team is uncertain whether the effect is caused by TURP or by differences in patient characteristics that we could not detect using the retrospective data available to us. The great majority of physicians do not believe the effect is due to the operation.

As a secondary strategy, however, there may be an advantage if practices not able to participate in randomized clinical trials (because open operations are not available) participate in preference trials. Under the hypothesis that patient differences do not account for the observed differences in mortality following TURP versus open prostatectomy, TURP appears to reduce life expectancy. The effect should therefore be observable in a preference trial where TURP is compared to a control population undergoing watchful waiting or some other alternative. An advantage of such preference trials would be the speed with which additional information on this important problem could be expected to emerge.

THE EVALUATIVE CLINICAL SCIENCES AND
THE FUTURE OF MEDICINE

I now turn to the more speculative task of attempting to relate outcomes research to current struggles about the future of medicine. Again, Thomas Kuhn provides an appropriate context. He teaches that when the rules and procedures of a science no longer deal effectively with anomalies of theory or experimental evidence, a new science emerges. Problems are stated in new ways; new disciplines establish themselves; and new techniques provide solutions not previously possible. I believe that the emergence of the evaluative clinical sciences, as a set of disciplines distinct from biomedical science, is a response to the increasingly obvious anomalies of the model on which clinical and health care policy decision making has been based. That model is the more or less passive delegation of decision making to physicians who, to use Kenneth Arrow's term, act as rational agents for patients and society to assure that health resources are distributed optimally. The rational agency theory depends on two key assumptions about physicians. First, that by virtue of the strength of biomedical science and their own clinical experience, physicians know the prognosis for the various treatments available to a patient with a given condition. Second, that physicians choose treatments that maximize patient utility, and that they can wisely choose the right treatment for the individual patient, disentangling their own preferences to deal with the problem of interpersonal differences in utility. This requires successful negotiation of E. B. White's observation that one man's meat is another man's poison, in order to make vicarious judgments about which treatment has the highest expected value for any patient.

The anomalies of rational agency theory are now evident to a widening audience. It is increasingly apparent that the large investment in biomedical science has not resulted in a consensus among physicians on the correct way to practice medicine, nor has it resulted in orderly assessment of treatment theories. Quite the contrary, biomedical science, by virtue of its prodigious success, appears to have increased uncertainty and practice-style variations by offering an ever increasing supply of new technology and new biomedical ideas. This is behind the shocking variations in costs and utilization between Boston and New Haven, where the scientific credentials of local medicine are state of the art. It is also increasingly apparent that patients want to participate in determining their own medical fates and that physicians have neither the information nor the decision making skills to always choose the treatment that will maximize patient utility. These challenges, emerging at a time of runaway costs, growing consumerism, and concern about patients' rights, have effectively dissolved long held assumptions about the efficacy, the ethical sufficiency, and the legal basis of the delegated decision making model.

The breakdown is apparent in two ways. On the microscale, the impact is felt in the changing doctor-patient relationship, where physicians face an increasingly assertive and sometimes litigious clientele. The passive trust that manifested itself in the patient's willingness to delegate decision making to the physician and accept what happens as fate has receded. More and more, patients demand active involvement in the decisions that determine their medical futures—even when this participation forces exposure to the reality that physicians do not know all the facts.

This is not to say that patients must distrust their physicians or that a significant minority now do. But it does identify a new relationship based on an active patient role where decision making is shared, not delegated. In this new role, the challenge to the physician is to learn how to function in what some have called the cognitive role—as an advisor or counselor who understands the need to act on imperfect information and who helps individual patients understand their own preferences, given the dilemmas the physician and the patient face together.

It is perhaps on the macroscale of socioeconomics, of reaction to runaway costs, that the breakdown is most acutely felt by physicians. Understanding the flaws in the rational agency theory helps explain runaway costs. Demand is not controlled by professional consensus on "correct practice"; the supply of manpower and technologies, medical theory and practice style, are in dynamic equilibrium. Technologic possibilities, the numbers of physicians practicing medicine, and the costs of care are now such that many politicians, government officials, corporate officers, and labor leaders perceive further growth in the health care sector as a threat to other societal priorities. More and more, government and private corporations are intruding into the doctor-patient relationship in their attempts to control demand.

The emergence of the evaluative clinical sciences and outcomes research is a response to the intellectual crisis created by the demise of the rational agency theory and the loss of faith that biomedical science, through its own internal logic, assures effective medical practice. It is an effort to provide the methodologies, strategies, and knowledge base needed to support a new model for clinical decision making, one that Albert Mulley has suggested be called the shared clinical decision making model. The model preserves the notion that consumer preferences and knowledge about outcomes should serve as the regulator of patient behavior and of aggregate demand. But it also recognizes the inherent limits in the ability of physicians to determine vicariously what treatments patients value most. The evaluative clinical sciences seek to make possible better clinical decisions based on a fuller understanding of outcome probabilities, and active participation of patients in selecting treatments.

The outcomes research agenda thus seeks to do something quite new. It focuses on the systematic evaluation of all of the outcomes that are relevant to patients—mortality, morbidity, complications, symptom reduction, and functional status improvement—as well as the physiologic or biochemical indicators which have perhaps too often been assumed to be valid surrogates for patient well-being. It focuses on the systematic evaluation of all (reasonably held) theories and alternative practice styles that are relevant to a particular condition or illness. It emphasizes assessment teams, organized around specific conditions with ongoing responsibility for evaluating all treatment options, old and new. The outcomes research agenda thus removes the "double standard of truth" that has characterized previous evaluation approaches. These approaches have mainly concentrated on new drug evaluations, while ignoring evaluations of the use of approved drugs in novel ways, of surgical operations and other procedures such as balloon angioplasty, or of the use of hospitals compared to ambulatory care settings for chronic and acute conditions. Outcomes research focuses on the development of methods and strategies for conveying information in ways that activate the patient as a partner in decision making. The research agenda includes a broad emphasis on learning to help patients make decisions consistent with their own preferences.

The outcomes research agenda focuses on new strategies and methods for making inferences to improve the validity and efficiency of evaluative research. Emphasis is placed on developing a proper balance between non-experimental and experimental methods for making inferences, and exploring the available options. Decision analysis is emphasized as a tool for organizing thinking, for conducting "thought experiments" to evaluate whether a particular treatment controversy is about the probabilities for outcomes, or whether it is really about the value of outcomes for patients. And, because the Shared Medical Decision

Making model emphasizes the importance of patient preferences, the agenda accentuates the need to learn the advantages and limitations of basing treatment assignments in prospective clinical research protocols on patient preference rather than on randomization.

REFERENCES

1. Wennberg JE, Bunker JP, Barnes B. The need for assessing the outcome of common medical practices. Annual Review of Public Health 1980;1:277–295.
2. American Medical Association. Confronting Regional Variations: The Maine Approach. Chicago: American Medical Association, 1986.
3. Wennberg JE, Freeman JL, Shelton RM, Bubolz TA. Hospital use and mortality among Medicare beneficiaries in Boston and New Haven. New England Journal of Medicine 1989;321:1168–1173.
4. Wennberg JE, Mulley AG, Hanley D et al. An assessment of prostatectomy for benign urinary tract obstruction. Journal of the American Medical Association 1988;259:3027–3030.
5. Fowler FJ, Wennberg JE, Timothy RP et al. Symptom status and quality of life following prostatectomy. Journal of the American Medical Association 1988;259:3018–3022.
6. Barry MJ, Mulley AG, Fowler FJ, Wennberg JE. Watchful waiting versus immediate transurethral resection for symptomatic prostatism. Journal of the American Medical Association 1988;259:3010–3017.
7. Wennberg J, Roos N, Sola L, Schori A, Jaffe R. Use of claims data systems to evaluate health care outcomes: Mortality and re-operation following prostatectomy. Journal of the American Medical Association 1987;257:933–936.

5

Strengths and Weaknesses of Health Insurance Data Systems for Assessing Outcomes*

LESLIE L. ROOS, NORALOU P. ROOS, ELLIOTT S. FISHER, and
THOMAS A. BUBOLZ

Health care data bases of varying scope and quality exist in a number of different settings: research groups, hospitals, insurers, and governmental agencies. Of particular interest are the data generated by health insurance systems in North America, Europe, Australia, and New Zealand. Because health care data collected for administrative purposes are evermore available and less expensive to analyze, it is not surprising that such data bases are increasingly used in·technology assessment and health policy research (1,2,3). Moreover, their use is explicitly advocated in the Patient Outcomes Research Team approach, established by the Agency for Health Care Policy and Research.

What kind of information from administrative data bases is useful for clinical analyses? Many American data bases, such as Medicare, commonly provide the following data from hospital discharge abstracts:

*Some of the material in this paper has appeared in: Roos LL, Sharp SM, Cohen MM, Wajda A. Risk adjustment in claims-based research: The search for efficient approaches. Journal of Clinical Epidemiology 1989;42:1193-1206; and Roos LL. Nonexperimental data systems in surgery. International Journal of Technology Assessment in Health Care 1989;5:341-386; and Rutkow IM (ed). Socioeconomics of Surgery. St. Louis: C.V. Mosby, 1989.

This paper was supported by the Institute of Medicine, by Career Scientist Awards from Health and Welfare, Canada (to Leslie L. Roos and Noralou P. Roos), and by grants from Health and Welfare, Canada (6607-1197-44) and from the National Center for Health Services Research (5 R18 HS-05745).

Patient-identifying information:
- Date of Birth
- Sex
- Place of Residence
- Identifying Number (individual or family)

Other items for analysis include:
- Discharge Diagnoses (several)
- Procedures Performed in Hospital (several)
- Hospital
- Date of Admission
- Date of Discharge
- Discharge Code (death, another hospital, home, etc.)

Secondary items include:
- Admitting Physician Identifying Number
- Physician Performing Each Procedure (identifying number)

Physician claims typically identify the patient, the service rendered, date of the service, and the physician. The major data bases are designed to describe patient characteristics, diagnoses, and treatments. One reason for incompleteness of data is that hospitals lack motivation to record information that does not have an immediate impact on reimbursement. An ideal data base would have the following characteristics:

- *System-wide coverage of an entire population.* Government-organized insurance systems are typically individual-based. Such coverage includes care received at a wide variety of institutions and from the whole universe of health care providers. Coverage of an entire population permits study of utilization from an epidemiologic perspective, attributing use to individuals according to place of residence, no matter where the services are provided. Subgroups or whole populations can be compared to see how much of any given resource is used. Such population-based data can be adjusted for age, sex, and other characteristics to facilitate comparisons.

- *Unique identifying number (or combination of identifiers).* When each person is identified in this manner, usage can be cumulated for each person, wherever care is received. This data base should record all contacts with the health care system for each individual, with the unique identifier available to facilitate tracing. Ideally, the data base would record all hospital care, both inpatient and outpatient, services in free-standing surgery centers, activities in physician offices, entry to nursing or personal care home, health care received at home, and prescription drug use. Thus, an individual having surgery in one setting who is readmitted to a second institution will have both contacts captured by the system.

- *Enrollment or registry file.* A file specifying when and why each individual's coverage begins and ends is very useful. Such a file is necessary to tell whether an individual with no recorded contact with the health care system resided in the jurisdiction and indeed had no contact; left the jurisdiction; or died. This type of file helps to determine the percentage of individuals enjoying intervention-free survival—survival without any contact with the health care system.

- *Comprehensiveness.* Data bases can be characterized by their comprehensiveness. Some aspects of comprehensiveness can determine the design of any study, from relatively simple to relatively complex. At the simplest level of administrative data bases (Level 3), only hospital discharge abstracts are needed (4). Level 3 data can support studies of length of stay and in-hospital mortality; when combined with coverage of a population, such information permits analyses of utilization across medical market areas. At the intermediate level, Level 2 data require consistent individual identifiers on hospital discharge abstracts. Hospital claims can be sorted by date and identifying number to generate hospitalization histories for each individual. Level 2 data can thus be used for short-term outcome studies of readmissions and complications after surgery. Such research on quality assurance and cost control can provide timely feedback to health care institutions. The most comprehensive Level 1 data bases possess all the features of the Level 2 and 3 files and include an enrollment file with dates for startup, death, and leaving the insurance plan. Longitudinal studies can follow individuals' health care utilization through time (see Table 5.1).

A Level 1 system offering complete coverage for a population can often provide large samples and impressive follow-up capabilities, whether the care be ambulatory, community, or hospital based. The proportion of individuals enjoying intervention-free survival can also be ascertained. The ability to develop individual longitudinal histories (before and after an event or index hospitalization) permits identifying first-time occurrences in a population. These incident cases present a more homogeneous group for study; a second operation or recurrence of a condition can be distinguished from new events. Alternative treatments and different hospitals can be compared and analyses carried out across medical market areas on a per-person basis.

STRENGTHS

System-Wide, Population-Based Data

System-wide coverage allows us to monitor the effectiveness of clinical treatments. Since administrative data bases are not limited to specific institutions, they include poor health outcomes which occur following discharge from an institution. This makes possible comparative studies of outcomes from institutions with very different lengths of stay. Because administrative data bases

TABLE 5.1 Data requirements and types of studies using hospital data

Data Requirements	Types of Studies

Simple—Level 3
Need hospital discharge
   abstracts
	In-hospital Mortality
	   Volume-outcome comparisons,
	     monitoring of individual hospitals
	Length of Stay
	Small-Area Analyses
	Changes over Time

Intermediate—Level 2
Need hospital discharge
   abstracts and consistent
   individual identifiers
	Timely Longitudinal Research
	Short-Term Readmissions
	Volume-Outcome Comparisons
	Monitoring of Individual Hospitals
	Quality Assurance and Cost Control

Comprehensive—Level 1
Need hospital discharge
   abstracts, consistent
   individual identifiers,
   and enrollment file
	Highest Quality Longitudinal Research
	Shortest-Term and Long-Term
	   Outcome Studies
	Identification of Incident Cases
	Volume-Outcome Comparisons
	Monitoring of Individual Hospitals
	Choice of Treatment
	Small-Area Analysis by Person

SOURCE: Rutkow IM (ed), Socioeconomics of Surgery. St. Louis: C. V. Mosby, 1989.

cover care received by multiple providers, complications which might not be picked up in any individual practice can be detected. For example, almost half (42.6 percent) the Manitoba surgeons performing repeat resections were not the physicians who had performed the original prostatectomies (5). Patients may not return to a physician if they are dissatisfied or have poor outcomes on a treatment he or she has prescribed; without system-wide follow-up, physicians may overestimate the positive aspects of their treatment.

Efficacy versus Effectiveness

This problem can be stated simply: treatments that produce excellent outcomes in a research setting (efficacious) may not be beneficial (effective) when applied to a different spectrum of patients in clinical situations. Community hospital practices and medical care outcomes may differ widely from those publicized by researchers at academic centers.

Research on efficacy of procedures or the results of the so-called "best" situation (generally a teaching hospital) are usually reported in studies of technology assessment (6). But technology assessment is not well developed; a lack of information on the efficacy of many procedures (7) may make physicians uncertain about choice of treatment (8).

The rarity of a condition (9) almost always presents problems in assessing efficacy by randomized clinical trials. Non-experimental research may show clinical trials to be "so difficult to organize or so costly as to be impractical" (10). Even when clinical trials have been performed, non-experimental data bases can play a valuable role. For example, population-oriented data bases facilitate long-term follow-up of clinical trials. Claims research can also help specify the relevance of clinical trials. If clinical trials have too stringent criteria for entry, actual physician practice may be so different that the results are only partially applicable.

Evaluation of quality of care in both types of settings can be made easier by population-based data, since studies of efficacy and effectiveness can use the same non-experimental data systems. Effectiveness studies that present outcome results from representative samples of all hospitals and all physicians are rare. Administrative data can be particularly valuable for such research.

Large Numbers and Time Series

An added benefit of the system-wide coverage characteristic of administrative data bases is the large numbers of cases and controls which can typically be identified. Administrative data bases help expand the number and type of outcomes traced. In other words, if the mortality rate is too low to permit a statistically strong analysis, we can study additional poor outcomes, including complications reflected in hospital readmissions and patterns of physician visits.

If there are insufficient cases in a given year, additional years can be examined. Thus, a population can be tracked over a longer period to accumulate enough events to permit analyses. This is especially useful with rare conditions, such as infective endocarditis (11).

Ongoing health insurance systems add a new set of observations every year. Potentially, analysts can go back to the beginning to find those items of information which are routinely recorded. These long series of data allow retrospective cohort studies. For example, in 1989 a researcher can go back to surgery cases recorded in 1979 and do a 10-year follow-up.

Long-term studies of health outcomes can give very different assessments of the efficacy of a given procedure. A workshop convened by the National Institutes of Health (12) suggested that after transurethral prostatectomy, "the need for further operative treatment is uncommon"; however, the cumulative eight-year probability of having a second operation was recently found to be 20.2 percent (13).

Administrative data can also be used before an event of interest to define incident cases. A study of infective endocarditis listed all Manitoba patients hospitalized with the condition from April 1, 1979, to March 31, 1985. Then "incident cases were identified by eliminating those individuals with previously diagnosed infective endocarditis in the April 1, 1976 - March 31, 1979 period" (11).

In similar fashion, data on histories can help create clean comparison groups. For example, in a study of whether tubal ligation increases a woman's risk of having a hysterectomy, Cohen (14) identified as her control group a random sample of women aged 25 to 44 and eliminated all individuals who had a hysterectomy prior to July 1974 or tubal ligation from 1970 through 1982.

The time series characteristics of data bases can also be used to characterize individuals by health care usage/morbidity patterns to develop measures of case-mix adjustment. This application of administrative data bases is treated in detail in the section on risk adjustment.

Events Unaffected by Recall

We know that patient reports of drug exposure, hospitalizations, physician visits, and medical conditions are subject to recall biases. Ray and Griffin (15) note that a primary "strength of Medicaid data for pharmacoepidemiology is the availability of detailed pharmacy records from which drug exposure history can be constructed." Most evidence suggests that events such as hospitalizations and physician visits are well recorded in health insurance systems. As discussed later, diagnoses recorded in the administrative data have limitations, which are often related to characteristics of medical practice; two physicians seeing the same patient will sometimes diagnose different entities. Overall, diagnoses recorded in the claims system are physician-originated and likely as accurate as patient self-reports.

Accurate recording of past health events is critical in developing lifetime estimates of an exposure (such as x-ray usage) or when timing of an event is important. Thus, in assessing the effectiveness of influenza vaccine, it is important to know whether the vaccine was delivered and if it was given during the appropriate period.

Unobtrusive Nature

A great advantage of administrative data is that they permit relatively unobtrusive research. Because studies using these data are done as statistical analyses, patient consent is not sought. There are no biases because persons refuse to participate or because patients, providers, or data collectors know about the study. This is important. The biases that arise when subjects know to which group they have been randomized, or even when participants know they are involved in a study, have been discussed elsewhere (16). Hertzman (17), for example, has shown that information on health status from an occupational group explicitly under study may differ from that obtained from a population unaware of the purpose of the study.

Multiple Comparisons

The fact that individuals are not randomly assigned to comparison groups raises questions as to the comparability of individuals and hospitals being studied. Such questions arise regardless of the method of risk adjustment—administrative data, chart review, physical examination, etc. Administrative data generally give several ways to test the consistency of findings after risk adjustment.

Hypotheses often can be tested among a number of subgroups in the population. In a recent study of prostatectomy, N. Roos et al. (2) found higher mortality among men having transurethral prostatectomies (the more accepted operation) than among those having open prostatectomies (the older operation). The risk-adjusted results from one Manitoba teaching hospital held for all men having prostatectomies and for a subgroup of the healthiest men. Testing across populations is also helpful. Comparisons using administrative data from four countries confirmed the findings of differential mortality after transurethral and open prostatectomies.

Statistical models can also be compared. When several covariates are available, a number of regression models can be tested for consistency. If relative risk of mortality or another dependent variable does not change as covariates are entered or deleted, faith in the findings is increased (18,19).

Design Flexibility

Researchers designing cohort and case-control studies must deal with critics, friendly and otherwise, who suggest changes in the design of their study. One great advantage of administrative data is design flexibility, the ability to alter a research design with little difficulty. For example, changes in definition of exposure may involve: (a) altering the time period during which an intervention (such as immunization for flu) is seen to be relevant, and (b) redefining control groups to make them parallel with the group receiving a treatment. The variables used for matching purposes can be easily changed. Finally, several designs can be used with the same administrative data base. For example, a planned study of the efficacy of influenza vaccination will utilize both cohort and case-control designs constructed from the Manitoba data base. Similar design flexibility should be possible using the Medicare data.

Potential for Multiple Projects

Because administrative data systems are not designed for specific studies, they can be valuable for multiple projects. For example, a set of files originally developed to examine the short-term outcomes associated with cholecystectomy were subsequently used in a study to develop computerized methods for monitoring readmissions following surgery, changes over time in quality of care over a 10-year period, quality of care, and health care outcomes in the native and non-native communities. More recently, the literature suggests there may be an elevated risk of heart disease following cholecystectomy; these files will again be reassessed.

The flip side of having a data set with the potential for multiple analyses is to be accused of being theoretical and opportunistic in one's research. Because health care data bases are not closely restricted in subject matter and because there are limits to the type of data they make available, studies should be tailored to their strengths. For example, coding systems do not identify laterality, so studying outcomes of procedures which can be performed only on one part of the body (prostatectomy) is much easier than studying conditions where a second procedure will not necessarily represent a complication but may be a new event (total hip replacement or cataracts).

Focus on Risks

Administrative data banks, by their focus on health care interventions, make possible more accurate assessment of risks associated with treatment (mortality; readmissions; specific sequelae such as prostate revisions, stricture dilations, etc.). Given the uncertainties surrounding major areas of medical treatment such as bypass surgery and carotid endarterectomy, it might be appropriate to concentrate on comparing the risks associated with new and established treatments until firm data on the benefits of medical treatment are developed.

Clinical Decision Making

Models of the clinical decision process must present choices the way clinicians do. These decisions may or may not require specific test results. Thus, the adequacy of administrative data for decision models depends on the condition and the procedure studied. Successful modeling has been carried out for medical versus surgical treatment of infective endocarditis (11) and for watchful waiting versus surgery for prostate disease (20).

The decision tree for modeling treatment of infective endocarditis highlights the usefulness of claims data. The data base provided estimates of the probabilities of a number of events after two strategies: early surgery or attempted medical cure. Variables used in the decision tree included probabilities of operative mortality, probabilities of events (including dying and congestive heart failure) before or soon after four weeks of antibiotic therapy, probabilities of events occurring long after completion of antibiotic therapy, and life expectancies in weeks under different treatment regimes.

WEAKNESSES

Structural Limitations

Administrative data sets generally allow the collection of a fixed amount of information on all events for all people covered by an insurance program. These data sets are designed to answer such questions as who receives treatment, when was the treatment given, where was the treatment given, who gave the treatment, what was the treatment, and how much did it cost.

Administrative data typically have structural limitations inherent in the record layout, available codes, and coding regulations. Such limitations can be overcome only through structural changes in either the record or the regulations. Several coding issues are of interest to the researcher. A single surgical procedure or hospitalization may result in a single hospital record and one or more physician bills. Linkage of the surgeon's claim to the hospital claim has been shown to be an excellent way to check on the reliability of the coding of hospital procedures.

At the same time, for many procedures and diagnoses, different codes may plausibly be used to describe the same event. One physician or insurance carrier may prefer a given code, while others use different codes. Because several physicians often submit bills for treating the same condition in the same patient (surgeon, assistant, anesthetist), there is a real possibility that different codes will be used. However, multiple bills for the same event offer another way to confirm the occurrence of events or test the reliability of the initial claim.

The precision of codes varies across conditions. For many conditions, the ICD-9-CM hospital codes, used in the Medicare and Manitoba data bases, and tariff codes, such as CPT, are highly precise in their specification of the procedure and the clinical problem. Examples include transurethral prostatectomy and carotid endarterectomy. Studying these conditions or treatments through the claims data is relatively straightforward.

Sometimes the tariff codes are more precise than the ICD-9-CM codes; this seems to be the case with hip repair procedures. Other procedures may be poorly classified on hospital and physician claims and may be more problematic to study; vascular surgery presents difficulties in this regard. Diagnoses generally are less precise than most researchers would prefer; "congestive heart failure" and "diabetes mellitus" encompass broad ranges of severity that may mask important clinical subgroups.

The detail of the coding conventions may be inadequate for some studies. The ICD-9-CM coding system does not distinguish procedures performed on the left side of the body from those done on the right side. This makes it more difficult to assess the results of orthopedic surgery; a second hip or knee replacement operation on someone who has already had one may mean either a reoperation or an operation on the other extremity (21).

Moreover, the data captured by administrative data systems may not be those of most interest to health outcome studies. While the data system may record the occurrence of certain events (laboratory tests, x-rays, pap smears, etc.), the results of these tests typically are not available in an administrative data system. In fact, before beginning a study with an administrative data bank, the key question is: "Can the event of interest be defined in the system and are key outcomes captured?" The answer depends on the specific recording systems used. It may be several years before a new procedure, such as angioplasty, is accurately recorded in this system.

Finally, the timing of diagnoses during a hospitalization cannot be determined from the discharge abstract alone. Consequently, conditions that develop in the course of treatment cannot be distinguished from comorbid conditions present at the time of admission—an important distinction for risk-adjusted outcome analyses (22,23). For example, Medicare patients who develop a pulmonary embolus after surgery cannot be reliably distinguished from those who had the condition before the operation. Other data systems (such as that in Manitoba) may be able to make this distinction by linking physician claims. Ongoing work is directed toward estimating the probability that such conditions will develop during surgical hospitalization for a number of procedures.

Bias Due to Reporting and Coding

There are several threats to the validity of claims data (24). The data submission process and coding of the data can lead to reporting and coding errors. However, financial incentives for providers to assure adequate reimbursement and for funding agencies to minimize expenditures provide some protection against lost or inaccurate data. Another source of bias is that contacts with the system generating the data have to be initiated by someone, often the patient. The probability of contact with the system may be affected by hospital and physician supply.

The accuracy of procedural and diagnostic data depends upon both the physicians and the clerks involved. American Medicare data appear to record procedures performed with fair accuracy, particularly if the "order of procedure" is ignored. Medicare data quality may have gone up since the introduction of the Prospective Payment System, but diagnostic information may not be as accurate as in the Manitoba files (25,26,27). Medicare data also do not include outpatient information in the hospital file. In Manitoba, both surgical procedures performed in hospitals and discrete billable items (even if not major events, including tests such as pap smears) appear to be reliably captured in the claims system.

The quality of diagnostic data also depends upon the source. Diagnoses on hospital records are likely to be more accurate than diagnoses on claims generated by physician's visits. In Manitoba, diagnoses are noted with a reasonable degree of accuracy and specificity in the hospital system, reflecting the professional training of medical records technicians. A comparison of diagnoses recorded on hospital records with those reported in the claims showed 95 percent correspondence in gallbladder disease, and 89 to 92 percent correspondence in a study of acute myocardial infarction (28,29).

Although Medicare does not include ambulatory care diagnoses with the physician claims, other data systems may contain this diagnostic information. Such diagnoses are useful at a more general level. One fruitful approach in Manitoba has been to group diagnoses available from physician claims (for example, contacts for gynecologic problems in a study of women undergoing hysterectomy, and gallbladder disease and abdominal pain for a study of contacts before and after gallbladder surgery) rather than to attempt fine diagnostic distinctions (25,30).

Bias Due to Differential Contact

As noted earlier, contact bias is a threat to the interpretation of claims data; the individual rather than the researcher generally initiates contact with the system generating the data. Thus, a person who is ill, but has no contact with the health care system, does not produce a record on this episode of illness or chronic condition. Such contact can be important for studying outcomes. For example, Manitoba research has used readmission to hospital in the three months after hysterectomy as an indication of post-surgical complications.

The probability of an individual contacting a physician or being hospitalized varies with certain system characteristics (such as insurance coverage and supply factors), individual characteristics (care-seeking behavior), and physician factors (propensity to hospitalize) (31). Given universal insurance, relatively few ill individuals lack contact with the health care system when the measurement period is several years (32). In the United States, however, co-payment is likely to accentuate contact bias. Poorly covered individuals may be precisely those who receive the poorest care; analyses thus may underestimate poor outcomes.

Supply factors are important and readily studied. Assuming similar insurance coverage for all members of a political unit, the supply of physicians and hospital beds has been shown to affect system usage (33). Supply variables have been shown to be statistically significant in predicting such outcomes as readmissions. Data on bed and physician supply per capita generally are fairly easy to obtain for different geographic units. By controlling for these factors on a small-area basis, analyses of readmissions and other utilization can continue in a statistically sound manner.

Benefits of Treatment

It is difficult to identify benefits of treatment in an administrative data system. Estimates of quality of life are very indirect. Changes in the frequency of diagnoses and hospitalization provide some information, and periods of intervention-free survival following a key event can be calculated. These variables may be unsatisfactory as a measure of real benefit of the procedure, although some studies show substantively significant relationships between utilization and morbidity (32,34).

CONTROVERSIAL AREAS

Risk Adjustment

Risk adjustment poses a major problem in evaluating outcomes across hospitals and physicians (35). If patients operated upon at Hospital A have higher mortality and complication rates than patients operated upon at Hospital B, is it because Hospital A's operating team is less skilled? Or is it because the case-mix of patients at the two institutions is different, with Hospital A treating higher-risk patients?

One issue with significant implications for studies of quality assurance and cost control is: when can claims data alone be used for these controls and when is prospective data collection necessary? What controls are good enough for testing hypotheses about the relationship between surgical volume and treatment outcomes, for distinguishing the better of two treatments, and for identifying hospitals or physicians with particularly poor or especially good outcomes?

The issue of how much additional information is provided per unit of cost is vital when expensive primary data collection is being considered. Researchers have assumed that the optimal approach would incorporate primary data collection, possibly combining clinical judgment with physiologic information and diagnostic testing (18,19,23). On the other hand, the ability of researchers and clinicians to predict the morbidity and mortality following medical and surgical treatment is clearly limited.

Figure 5.1 illustrates our view of the utility of information. The variation explained is presented on the Y axis, while the X axis measures effort. The predictive power provided by better algorithms applied to a given data type reaches a "flat of the curve" situation fairly quickly. Figure 5.1 suggests the greater predictive power of the first covariates in a multivariate analysis. If primary data are collected, they may well be among the best predictors (36). But when several measures are available, they are largely substitutable for each other.

One promising taxonomy for comorbidity takes into account not only the number but also the seriousness of comorbid diseases. The comorbidity index of Charlson et al. (37) explained a higher proportion of the variance in one-year

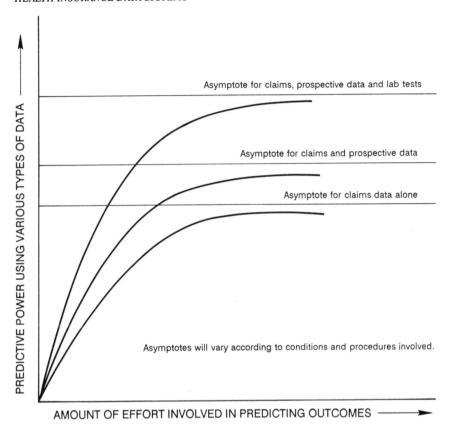

FIGURE 5.1 Analytical effort involved to produce results for different types of data. Asymptotes will vary according to conditions and procedures involved. SOURCE: Roos LL, Sharp SM, Cohen MM, Wajda A. Risk adjustment in claims-based research: The search for efficient approaches. Journal of Clinical Epidemiology 1989;42:1193–1206.

survival rates than a model based solely on the number of comorbid diseases. In a test population with a large set of clinical and demographic variables, age and the comorbidity index were found to be the only significant predictors of death attributable to comorbid disease. This index has been used in a number of claims-based studies (2,18,19).

Computerized hospital admission/separation abstracts can be used to generate covariates, such as the Charlson comorbidity index, for risk adjustment. In assessments done in Manitoba, the addition of other sorts of information (claims from physician visits, health status indices from surveys, and even some prospectively collected clinical data) generated little additional power in predicting hospitalization, nursing home entry, and mortality (19,38).

Manitoba Level 3 data (from the surgical event alone) using age, sex, and limited comorbidity information have provided almost as good risk adjustment in predicting mortality and post-surgical readmissions as Level 1 data (from the history of hospitalizations in the preceding six months and the surgical event). A model using only prognostic data (comorbidity information from the computerized history preceding surgery) also resulted in fairly good risk adjustment and similar overall results. Thus, Blumberg's (22) concerns about using information from the index hospitalization, rather than prognostic data, do not seem critical.

Considerable progress in adjusting for risk by chart review has also been made. Daley et al. (23) have built upon the APACHE II system to develop a chart-based clinical risk adjustment system, the Medicare Mortality Predictor System, to predict hospital mortality. However, when researchers using inexpensive nonintrusive measures such as claims must decide whether to invest scarce resources in more data collection, they must evaluate the likely yield of the additional information (39). It is difficult to find the proper point or points between "gold standard" technology assessment research that relies on extensive primary data collection and somewhat less accurate but cheaper and more timely approaches. We need research to compare the power of additional chart review with claims-based work. Direct comparisons of predictive power and biases would define whether widespread additional data gathering is cost effective in risk adjustment.

If cross-sectional data can accurately identify patients at different degrees of risk, large-scale studies of in-hospital mortality following surgery become relatively easy to conduct. The literature comparing outcomes across institutions is buttressed by research supporting the validity of controls generated by cross-sectional data (40,41). Claims-based research certainly suggests that useful general covariates can be produced; different covariates need not necessarily be generated for each treatment or condition studied (19,36).

Outcome Measures

Some outcome measures require labor-intensive data collection through patient interviews or hospital records review. On the other hand, administrative data, such as insurance claims, provide an excellent source for nonintrusive measures such as readmissions and mortality. Because many data bases are maintained and updated for administrative purposes, analyses can be done for a relatively small marginal cost.

Most of our knowledge about variation in outcomes is derived from studies using nonintrusive measures. Such measures can be particularly valuable in screening large data bases "to flag events and caregivers with suspect profiles of performance" (42). Death is easily documented, usually from multiple sources such as death certificates, hospital reports, and insurance claims. However, as mortality rates decline, the number of deaths, particularly following single procedures or treatments, becomes very small. Thus, the study of non-fatal events (morbidity) and effects on quality of life has become more important in recent years. "Intervention-free survival" has been useful for studying surgical outcomes, and claims data might also be used to measure remission-free years for chronic diseases. Other nonintrusive measures based on claims data are important here:

1. Short-term readmission to hospital, within a specified period after surgery and for post-surgical complications. Building on previous work (43), panels of specialists, meeting under the auspices of the Health Care Financing Administration (HFCA), have developed lists of reasons for readmission, which indicate possible complications after a number of common procedures;

2. Additional surgery after the initial operation;

3. Long-term problems leading to hospital readmission, such as myocardial infarction and stroke; and

4. Subsequent physician visits with diagnoses indicating continuing problems.

Survey measures have been widely used. Their strength is the information they provide on attitudes, feelings, and tradeoffs; their weakness has been the cost of data collection (44). Self-perceived health, ability to perform activities of daily living, and ability to live independently in the community also are important for assessing health status. Finally, outcome studies focusing on providers generally emphasize patient satisfaction and physician performance standards.

EXPANDING DATA BASES

Record Linkage

Record linkage—the combining of separate records of the same individual—is a powerful new research tool. Linking specialized data bases with multipurpose claims data presents many research options, greatly increasing the amount and quality of data on individuals. Such capabilities are important because, no matter how much is recorded in any data base, specific items desired for a given study may not be available. Linkage can help make clinicians more comfortable with using administrative data; an expanded amount of information can provide many of the details clinicians associate with the practice of medicine. Record linkage helps deal with questions like: Does a given data set have enough detail to support research on efficacy and effectiveness? Are the data accurate and complete enough, and suitable for the purposes to which they are put?

Additional information may be contained in other sources which permit linkage to an existing data base. In particular, administrative data bases often do not include certain tests or x-rays if they are not billable, and the results of tests frequently are not included. Information on medical treatment (such as drugs used) typically is not available, making it difficult to compare medical and surgical alternatives for treatment of many conditions.

Although linkages involving Medicare claims typically use Social Security number, record linkage may involve files where these numbers, as well as name and address, are not available. Record linkage depends on having a sufficient number of identifiers of adequate power. Some relevant applications of record linkage are listed; the previously mentioned prostatectomy research used the first four linkages to help the Manitoba data base reach its potential (2):

1. Linkage of enrollment files or registries with Vital Statistics files to verify deaths and provide cause-of-death information. Given appropriate confidentiality safeguards, both Canadian and American governments cooperate with requests for death matching. These linkages underlie several longitudinal studies using Canadian and/or American data (45).

2. Linkage of claims with independently collected data from cancer registries to provide higher-quality information on the occurrence and date of diagnosis of cancer, thereby facilitating better case-mix controls, validity checks, and the potential for important independent studies (46).

3. Linkage of hospital and Vital Statistics information with preoperative data collected by one hospital's Anesthesia Quality Assurance Program produced a very rich data set on preoperative status of patients and operative outcomes (47). These data can help assess the efficacy of a number of surgical procedures by providing covariates (particularly the widely used American Society of Anesthesiologists' Physical Status score) to increase the credibility of claims-based analyses.

4. Linkage of hospital claims with physician claims to verify fact and date of surgery. These methods have supported extensive quality checks in Manitoba and are also being used with American Medicare data.

5. Linkage of survey information and claims to provide a fuller picture of the relationships among functional status, self-reported health status, and surgical outcomes (38). In Manitoba, linkage of two surveys of the aged may permit incorporation of the data into studies of procedures frequently done on the elderly.

Although the specific linkage keys differ in each example, the expanded files have supported a diverse set of studies. These types of linkage dramatically increase the amount and quality of individual-level data. Such an approach helps connect the perspective of the clinical epidemiologist and that of the health services researcher. Specialized data bases can be combined as appropriate with multipurpose claims data. Claims and detailed data from other sources can be put side by side to better understand the strengths and weaknesses of each.

Record linkage is a very valuable capability for researchers using non-experimental data. The mathematical concepts may be unfamiliar initially, but introductory texts and user-friendly software facilitate record linkage (45,48). A considerable amount of literature examines long-term mortality due to particular occupational health risks and provides examples of linkage studies in another context (45,49).

Primary Data Collection

What role does primary data collection play in claims-based research? We can specify cases which need futher checking when individual identifiers are available in administrative data sets. One purpose of primary data collection is to add detail on diagnosis or procedure. The importance of this added detail depends on the condition and procedure studied. For example, we may want to know the number of diseased vessels for research on coronary artery disease. We need information on laterality for studies of hip fractures; one needs to know if a second operation resulted from a complication or was a new procedure.

Primary data collection, particularly chart review, can also be used to confirm and buttress results obtained from analysis of administrative data bases. Such work can increase the clinical credibility of studies based on claims; for example, Malenka et al. (18) have reviewed Manitoba prostatectomies from one teaching hospital, generating comorbidity indices by independent chart review. The results, comparing outcomes of transurethral versus open prostatectomies, were similar to those produced from claims analyses (2).

Studies whose primary focus is collection of new information may still depend on claims data to identify patients or providers and to trace outcomes. Thus, the monitoring of hospital mortality, as done by HCFA, can help select hospitals for primary data collection. Primary data collection within the hospital can be facilitated by claims data which identify individuals, by name or number, whose charts should be pulled (18).

A fruitful way to combine methods is to use administrative data to identify individuals with a surgical treatment of interest; interviews could then examine satisfaction, subjective health status, quality of life, and so forth. Not only can claims data be used to identify specific cases but the linked data set can also generate information on outcomes (18). Similarly, studies of the appropriateness of care (50,51) might find it valuable to trace outcomes using enrollment files and claims data.

Combining administrative data and clinical data bases can compensate for weaknesses in claims data. For example, a proposed study of angina has isolated several problems with the claims and suggested ways to deal with these difficulties (see table on next page):

Limitations of Claims	Ways to Handle
Difficulty in distinguishing between stable and unstable angina using coding on hospital claims (discharge abstracts).	Linkage between hospital claims and more detailed clinical data will permit sensitivity testing of the importance of the stable versus unstable distinction.
In-hospital investigations will not generally appear on discharge abstracts.	Many tests are billable and will appear on physician claims. Chart review may be necessary to identify the others.
Information on some risk factors (smoking) and treatments (medical therapy) not available.	This information can be obtained from clinical data base.

Several valuable data bases obtained by extensive chart review are available for exploring what can and cannot be done using Medicare data. The largest linked Medicare data set seems to be that supplemented with data on Key Clinical Findings from eight Peer Review Organizations in seven states. As described elsewhere (52), the data were obtained from the medical record by a modification of the MedisGroups abstraction technique. Reviewers scan the record of the hospitalization and encode abnormalities in admission symptoms, history, the results of preadmission tests if documented in the medical record, physical examinations (including vital signs), and laboratory and specialized diagnostic tests. An extensive array of ICD-9-CM diagnostic codes (up to 30) and procedure codes (up to 36) is also recorded, as are untoward events in the course of the hospitalization.

DISCUSSION

Administrative data are rich in information that researchers should learn to use effectively. Research has generated questions about specific issues, such as the use of claims data to study medical treatments. Other issues are organizational and technical. Because outcomes research is interdisciplinary, we must develop ways to facilitate research across centers. Because it takes considerable cost and effort to organize administrative data for research purposes, we also need efficient information management.

Other questions relate to data needs: What constitutes clinically relevant information on claims data? What auxiliary information should be collected?

Technical questions include: How good are the linkages that tie health care data from different sources? How should individual records be organized? How should cleaning and checking be carried out? Current collaborations among a number of centers and researchers are posing and answering such questions.

REFERENCES

1. Jencks SF, Kay T. Do frail, disabled, poor, and very old Medicare beneficiaries have higher hospital charges? Journal of the American Medical Association 1987;257:198–202.
2. Roos NP, Wennberg JE, Malenka D, McPherson K, Anderson T, Cohen MM, Ramsey E. Mortality and reoperation following open and transurethral resection of the prostate for benign prostatic hypertrophy. New England Journal of Medicine 1989;320:1120–1124.
3. Roper WL, Winkenwerder W, Hackbarth GM, Krakauer H. Effectiveness in health care: An initiative to evaluate and improve medical practice. New England Journal of Medicine 1988;319:1197–1202.
4. Roos LL, Roos NP. Using large data bases for research on surgery. In Rutkow IM (ed). Socioeconomics of Surgery. St. Louis: C.V. Mosby, 1989:259–275.
5. Roos NP, Ramsey E. A population-based study of prostatectomy: Long term outcomes associated with differing surgical approaches. Journal of Urology 1987;137:1184–1188.
6. Brook RH, Lohr KN. Efficacy, effectiveness, variations, and quality: Boundary-crossing research. Medical Care 1985;23:710–722.
7. Patricelli RE. Employers as managers of risk, cost, and quality. Health Affairs 1987;6:75–81.
8. Wennberg JE. Improving the medical decision-making process. Health Affairs 1988;7:99–106.
9. Peto R. What treatments for rheumatoid arthritis can best be assessed by large, simple, long-term trials? British Journal of Rheumatology 1983;22:3–8.
10. Wennberg JE, Mulley AG, Hanley D, Timothy RP, Fowler FJ, Roos NP, Barry MJ, McPherson K, Greenberg ER, Soule D, Bubolz T, Fisher E, Malenka D. An assessment of prostatectomy for benign urinary tract obstruction: Geographic variations and the evaluation of medical care outcomes. Journal of the American Medical Association 1988;259:3027–3030.
11. Abrams HB, Detsky AS, Roos LL, Wajda A. Is there a role for surgery in the acute management of infective endocarditis? A decision analysis and medical database approach. Medical Decision Making 1988;8:165–174.
12. Grayhack JT, Sadlowski RW. Results of surgical treatment of benign prostatic hyperplasia. In Grayhack, Wilson, Scherbenske (eds). Benign Prostatic Hyperplasia, DHEW Publication No. NIH 76-1113, 1975:125–134. A workshop sponsored by the Kidney Disease and Urology Program of the National Institute of Arthritis, Metabolism and Digestive Diseases, National Institutes of Health.
13. Wennberg JE, Roos NP, Sola L, Schori A, Jaffe R. Use of claims data systems to evaluate health care outcomes: Mortality and reoperation following prostatectomy. Journal of the American Medical Association 1987;257:933–936.

14. Cohen MM. Long-term risk of hysterectomy after tubal sterilization. American Journal of Epidemiology 1987;125:410–419.
15. Ray WA, Griffin MR. Use of Medicaid data for pharmacoepidemiology. American Journal of Epidemiology 1989;129:837–849.
16. Kramer MS, Shapiro SH. Scientific challenges in the application of randomized trials. Journal of the American Medical Association 1984;252:2739–2745.
17. Hertzman C. Morbidity studies: Are population-based data a useful benchmark for studying morbidity in special groups? Canadian Journal of Public Health 1988;79:386–387.
18. Malenka DJ, Roos NP, Fisher ES, McLerran DF, Whaley FS, Barry MJ, Bruskewitz R, Wennberg J. Further study of the increased mortality following transurethral prostatectomy: A chart-based analysis. Journal of Urology in press.
19. Roos LL, Sharp SM, Cohen MM, Wajda A. Risk adjustment in claims-based research: The search for efficient approaches. Journal of Clinical Epidemiology 1989;42:1193–1206.
20. Barry MJ, Mulley AG, Fowler FJ, Wennberg JE. Watchful waiting vs. immediate transurethral resection for symptomatic prostatism: The importance of patients' preferences. Journal of the American Medical Association 1988;259:3010–3017.
21. Roos NP, Lyttle D. Hip arthroplasty surgery in Manitoba: 1973–1978. Clinical Orthopaedics 1985;199:248–255.
22. Blumberg MS. Risk adjusting health care outcomes: A methodologic review. Medical Care Review 1986;43:351–393.
23. Daley J, Jencks S, Draper D, Lenhart G, Thomas N, Walker J. Predicting hospital-associated mortality for Medicare patients: A method for patients with stroke, pneumonia, acute myocardial infarction, and congestive heart failure. Journal of the American Medical Association 1988;260:3617–3624.
24. Cook TD, Campbell DT. Quasi-Experimentation. Chicago: Rand McNally, 1979.
25. Demlo LK, Campbell PM. Improving hospital discharge data: Lessons from the National Hospital Discharge Survey. Medical Care 1981;19:1030–1040.
26. Hsia DC, Krushat WM, Fagan AB, Tebbutt JA, Kusserow RP. Accuracy of diagnostic coding for Medicare patients under the prospective-payment system. New England Journal of Medicine 1988;318:352–355.
27. Roos LL, Sharp SM, Wajda A. Assessing data quality: A computerized approach. Social Science and Medicine 1989;28:175–182.
28. Roos LL, Nicol JP, Johnson C, Roos NP. Using administrative data banks for research and evaluation: A case study. Evaluation Quarterly 1979;3:236–255.
29. Roos LL, Roos NP, Cageorge SM, Nicol JP. How good are the data? Reliability of one health care data bank. Medical Care 1982;20:266–276.
30. Davis H. Was surgery needed? The Baltimore Sun: April 6, 1986.
31. Roos NP, Flowerdew G, Wajda A, Tate RB. Variations in physicians' hospitalization practices: A population-based study in Manitoba, Canada. American Journal of Public Health 1986;76:45–51.
32. Mossey JM, Roos LL. Using insurance claims to measure health status: The illness scale. Journal of Chronic Diseases (Suppl 1) 1987;40:41S–50S.
33. Roos NP, Wennberg JE, McPherson K. Using diagnosis-related groups for studying variations in hospital admissions. Health Care Financing Review 1988;9:53–62.
34. Diaz C, Starfield B, Holtzman N, Mellits ED, Hankin J, Smalky K, Benson P. Ill

health and use of medical care: Community-based assessment of morbidity in children. Medical Care 1986;24:848–856.

35. Sloan FA, Perrin JM, Valvona J. In-hospital mortality of surgical patients: Is there an empiric basis for standard setting? Surgery 1986;99:446–453.

36. Flood AB, Scott WR. Hospital Structure and Performance. Baltimore: Johns Hopkins University Press, 1987.

37. Charlson ME, Pompei P, Ales KL, MacKenzie CR. A new method of classifying prognostic comorbidity in longitudinal studies: Development and validation. Journal of Chronic Diseases 1987;40:373–383.

38. Roos NP, Roos LL, Mossey JM, Havens BJ. Using administrative data to predict important health outcomes: Entry to hospital, nursing home, and death. Medical Care 1988;26:221–239.

39. Harrell FE, Califf RM, Pryor DB, Lee KL, Rosati RA. Evaluating the yield of medical tests. Journal of the American Medical Association 1982;247:2543–2546.

40. Showstack JA, Rosenfeld KE, Garnick DW, Luft HS, Schaffarzick RW, Fowles J. Association of volume with outcome of coronary artery bypass graft surgery: Scheduled vs. nonscheduled operations. Journal of the American Medical Association 1987;257:785–789.

41. U.S. Congress, Office of Technology Assessment. The Quality of Medical Care: Information for Consumers, OTA-H-386. Washington, D.C.: Government Printing Office, June 1988.

42. Berwick DM. Toward an applied technology for quality measurement in health care. Medical Decision Making 1988;8:253–258.

43. Roos LL, Cageorge SM, Austen E, Lohr KN. Using computers to identify complications after surgery. American Journal of Public Health 1985;75:1288–1295.

44. Fowler FJ, Wennberg JE, Timothy RP, Barry MJ, Mulley AG, Hanley D. Symptom status and the quality of life following prostatectomy. Journal of the American Medical Association 1988;259:3018–3022.

45. Newcombe HB. Handbook of Record Linkage. New York: Oxford University Press, 1988.

46. Cohen MM, Hammarstrand KM. Papanicolaou testing without a cytology registry. American Journal of Epidemiology 1989;129:388–394.

47. Cohen MM, Duncan PG. Physical status score and trends in anesthetic complications. Journal of Clinical Epidemiology 1988;41:83–90.

48. Wajda A, Roos LL. Simplifying record linkage: Software and strategy. Computers in Biology and Medicine 1987;17:239–248.

49. Smith ME. Record linkage: Organizing the facts together. In Bennett BM, Trute B (eds). Mental Health Information Systems: Problems and Prospects. New York: Edwin Mellen Press, 1984:263–281.

50. Winslow CM, Kosecoff JB, Chassin M, Kanouse DE, Brook RH. The appropriateness of performing coronary artery bypass surgery. Journal of the American Medical Association 1988;260:505–509.

51. Winslow CM, Solomon DH, Chassin MR, Kosecoff J, Merrick NJ, Brook RH. The appropriateness of carotid endarterectomy. New England Journal of Medicine 1988;318:722–727.

52. Krakauer H. The use of data abstracted from medical records to assess the effectiveness of medical interventions. Manuscript, 1988.

6

Prescription-Event Monitoring: An Example of Total Population Post-Marketing Drug Surveillance

WILLIAM H. W. INMAN

In the early 1970s in the United Kingdom, many patients who had been treated for heart disease with the beta-adrenergic blocking drug, practolol, suffered severe ocular and skin reactions and occasionally deafness or intestinal obstruction. Although these events were to be found in the patients' medical records, most of their physicians had failed to consider the possibility of a causal link with practolol and had no reason to report the cases to the Committee on Safety of Medicines (CSM). The need to supplement the yellow card scheme for voluntary reporting of suspected adverse reactions to drugs with a second scheme for recording events, irrespective of any recognized link with the use of new drugs, led to the establishment in 1980 of the United Kingdom's second national scheme, Prescription-Event Monitoring (PEM). This scheme was developed by the Drug Safety Research Unit (DSRU) in association with the University of Southampton.

"THE NUMBERS GAME"

Before describing PEM, it is worth reflecting on what can be described as "the numbers game." In Figure 6.1, I have attempted to indicate a number of variables which must be considered. The arrow at the bottom of the diagram represents the *severity* of an illness or symptom, ranging from trivial on the left to serious or life-threatening on the right. Above this is an arrow suggesting that, as severity increases, the *acceptable level of risk* of treatment may also increase from very low levels for a trivial complaint to much higher levels in the treatment of a serious or fatal illness.

Paradoxically, as the acceptable risk level rises the number of patients

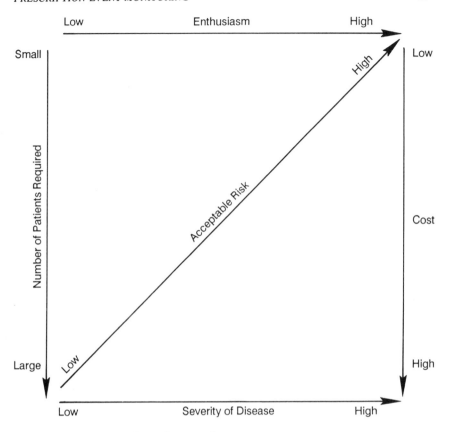

FIGURE 6.1 Variables in "the numbers game."

required to detect or measure it and the cost of the study diminish. Very large risks (e.g., 1 in 10) can be measured in comparatively small numbers of patients (e.g., 100) at relatively low cost. On the other hand, to measure the acceptable level of risk of mortality for symptomatic treatment of a headache, which may be less than 1 in 1 million, would require huge numbers of patients and infinite resources. Unfortunately, nobody has ever been able to tell us precisely what is an acceptable level of risk for a particular treatment. If the authorities were able to define a risk level which would lead them to remove a drug from the market, people like myself would be better able to design appropriate studies and estimate their cost.

I have added another variable at the top of the diagram to suggest a factor which people frequently forget. This is *enthusiasm*, which ranges from little or none for studies of very minute risks to considerable enthusiasm for studying large risks associated with the treatment of very serious diseases such as cancer.

I could have added yet another dimension to the diagram, which is *time*. It is worth remembering that some adverse effects of drugs might not become manifest for many years (e.g., carcinogenesis). Time adds to the costs of studies and also diminishes the enthusiasm of people to undertake them. Few people of my age, for example, would be keen to commence a carcinogenicity study, the results of which might be submitted to the *New England Journal of Medicine* by my grandson.

Clinical trials in 2,000-3,000 patients are likely to measure only the comparatively large risks associated with treatment of the more serious illnesses. They have the advantages of comparatively low cost and high enthusiasm of those involved. At the other extreme, voluntary reporting is the only practical and affordable way to detect very rare events. There is no way that any nation can afford to set up post-marketing studies capable of measuring risks in the region of 1 in 1 million or less. Even if every detail of patient care were recorded electronically for the whole population, the numbers and time involved in collecting sufficient data to be sure that a headache treatment was safe would be prohibitive. Somewhere between these two extremes, between the clinical trial on the one hand and voluntary reporting on the other, are a number of schemes aimed at measuring middle-level risks, those in the region of 1 in 100 to 1 in 10,000.

VOLUNTARY REPORTING SYSTEMS

From 1964 to 1980, I was responsible for managing CSM's yellow card reporting scheme in the United Kingdom, which is very similar to the voluntary reporting scheme operated by the Food and Drug Administration in the United States. I believe that, while voluntary reporting is the only practicable way to identify very rare or unusual events, we must be careful about using data derived from voluntary reports as the sole basis for decision making, particularly when the events are fairly common. Gastrointestinal hemorrhage associated with the use of non-steroidal anti-inflammatory drugs (NSAIDs) is a good example of a fairly common event. Each year, it occurs in between 1 in 1,000 and 1 in 200 people of an age commonly associated with arthritis or rheumatism, even in the absence of treatment with an NSAID. For this kind of event, it is always necessary to seek measurements of incidences from other types of study.

In 1976 I described the "seven deadly sins" of reporting doctors (1). First is the complacent belief that only safe drugs are marketed. Next is fear of litigation. Third, feelings of guilt about having done something for the benefit of the patient which has gone wrong. Fourth, and perhaps worst of the deadly sins, is an ambition to collect and publish a personal series of cases. It may be nice to see one's name in print, but it is not good to keep quiet about early observations and thereby delay general recognition of an important hazard. Fifth is ignorance of the need for reporting or of the reporting mechanism. Sixth is diffidence about deciding whether or not an event is an adverse drug reaction or something which would occur spontaneously, tinged perhaps with concern about appearing ignorant to those to whom the event would be reported. Finally, the seventh sin is old-fashioned lethargy. All seven deadly sins may have worked in producing the practolol disaster in my country, which led to blindness and a number of deaths. In that disaster it was estimated that 100,000 patients had been treated for a year or more before a single yellow card report of conjunctivitis reached the CSM (2).

POST-MARKETING SURVEILLANCE

In 1976 I proposed a scheme known as "recorded release," which would use our unique ability in the United Kingdom to assemble all prescriptions written under the National Health Service (1). This scheme and a number of later variants, such as "retrospective assessment of drug safety," were all turned down on the grounds of impracticality by those who advised the ministers of the day. After four years of negotiations with the various bodies concerned with the ethics of what has become known as pharmacoepidemiology, and particularly with issues of confidentiality and patient consent, I set up the DSRU within the faculty of medicine at the University of Southampton in June 1980. Our first PEM study commenced in 1981. Since that time our staff has increased from three to nearly fifty. In 1986, for a number of administrative and financial reasons, the management of the DSRU was transferred from the university to a charitable trust known as the Drug Safety Research Trust.

Because no one can predict which drug will be the next practolol, the only sensible policy is to study all new chemical entities marketed on a wide scale in general practice. We depend to a considerable extent on the drug industry for support, but we like to do the work first and hope that we will be reimbursed realistically after we have completed the study. The DSRU does not undertake contract work. Our staff are not allowed to receive regular retainers and may not hold shares in drug companies. We do not offer payment to doctors prior to their writing a drug prescription, and thus we do not in any way influence their selection of patients for treatment.

PRESCRIPTION-EVENT MONITORING

Prescription-Event Monitoring is based on the unique facility provided by the Prescription Pricing Authority (PPA) in the United Kingdom. All National Health Service prescriptions issued by general practitioners find their way to this central agency so that pharmacists can be remunerated. This facility has been available for more than 40 years, but only in 1980 was it possible to get agreement to use prescriptions, which are highly confidential documents, to identify very large cohorts of patients for epidemiological study (3).

PEM is conducted only in England, in a study population approaching 50 million patients because, in Wales particularly but also in Scotland and Northern

Ireland, large numbers of patients share the same name. An individual is often extremely difficult to identify from the limited details shown on the prescription. In England some 350 million prescriptions are written each year, and the PPA employs approximately 2,000 clerical staff who each process about 100 prescriptions per hour. Patients are not identified in the PPA data base. To identify them for research purposes, the PPA has to prepare a computer-generated "picking list" for each new chemical identity on our PEM list. The prescriptions are then pulled out of the files by hand and photocopied for transmission to the DSRU; up to 1 million prescriptions are handled each year for the purpose of PEM.

Let us briefly consider the word "event." Event monitoring was the idea of professor David Finney, who is currently a trustee of the DRSU and a founding member of the Adverse Reactions Subcommittee of the CSM. Finney pointed out that if you ask doctors to report "events," without worrying whether they are drug related, you may get a great deal more information. An "event" includes any new diagnosis, any reason for referring a patient to a hospital, any unexpected improvement in a patient's condition, any change of treatment, any suspected adverse reaction or indeed any significant word which a doctor has thought important enough to record in a patient's notes. Each of the questionnaires that we use to obtain clinical information from the general practitioner carries a very simple example: a broken leg is undoubtedly an "event." If we were comparing three drugs used for the same disease, and found that patients treated with drug B suffered four or five times as many fractures as those treated with A or C, we might suspect that we had a problem with hypotension, dizziness, or even softening of the bones. This simple concept of an event has been communicated to more than 20,000 general practitioners who participate enthusiastically. An important aspect of event monitoring is that, because the reporting of an event does not require a medical opinion as to its cause, it may well carry considerably less medico-legal risk than reporting an adverse reaction. An adverse reaction, after all, is an admission that something has gone wrong as a direct consequence of the physicians's decision to advise use of the drug.

Routinely, as soon as a new chemical entity is marketed for use in general practice we inform the PPA. In due course, increasingly large numbers of photocopied prescriptions are sent to the DSRU. We process them on our computer and after an interval that depends on the type of drug being studied, we post our questionnaires (green forms) to the doctors. We expect a response of about 70 percent.

The DSRU has a comprehensive system for following up individual case reports. All deaths are followed up. With the doctor's permission we contact the Family Practitioner Committee, to whom the notes usually have been returned after the patient's death. We are thus able to study the lifetime medical records of each patient who has died. Similarly, a non-fatal but serious event will be followed up by reference to a physician or surgeon at the hospital. We also obtain copies of all death certificates from the Office of Population Censuses and Surveys (OPCS), and have developed but not yet used a flagging technique to identify cohorts of patients through the OPCS so that we would be notified of any patient deaths. This process could be used for long-term monitoring of efficacy and serious problems such as carcinogenicity. Occasionally we have "banked" large numbers of prescriptions without taking any further action, so that, if a problem should arise 10 or 15 years later, a population is available for retrospective research.

During the last year or so we have experimented with a "red alert scheme." In collaboration with the CSM we issued a special variant of the yellow card on receipt of each prescription identifying a new patient. On the whole the scheme proved unsatisfactory. Many doctors were confused about what should be reported on the new yellow card. Although they were instructed to keep the card in the patient's notes and to use it only on the rare occasions when a serious or life-threatening adverse reaction occurred, large numbers of cards came back reporting that nothing had gone wrong or describing trivial events. We have now substituted a two-track system. A conventional green form is sent to the doctor within about three months of writing the first prescription. Then, where necessary, we return the same form one or two years later for an update.

The expanding data base offers all sorts of opportunities for outside research workers. For example, we are running an exercise with the help of the Merck Foundation which checks the results of our own follow-up of deaths with what has been written on the death certificate. Some very interesting differences are obvious. For example, if one believes what is written on death certificates, one might think there is almost no risk of dying from open heart surgery. Deaths tend to be due to less exciting causes, such as bronchopneumonia, which in some cases appears to develop before the patient has left the operating room!

We attempt to study all new chemical entities in addition to any older drug which may have caused problems. There are some exclusions. We do not routinely look at parenteral preparations because they are not generally used on a sufficiently wide scale by general practitioners. At the moment we do not study vaccines or topical preparations. So many new chemical entities are being released for marketing that the resources of the PPA and the capacity of our computer are somewhat stretched. For each drug we attempt to select about 20,000 patients, with the objective of an absolute minimum of 10,000 well-documented cases at the end of each study. To date, we have completed 11 studies. We abandoned 6 others because the drugs did not sell and we could not build up a worthwhile cohort over a period of three or four years. A drug which is slow to penetrate the market can cause a great deal of additional work because the ratio of repeat prescriptions to new patient identifications is large. Currently we have more than 20 studies in progress and 5 or 6 others in the pipeline.

PEM has occasionally been used to test hypotheses. For example, we looked into erythromycin estolate because yellow card reporting suggested the possibility that the estolate was relatively more likely to cause jaundice than other forms of erythromycin. A comparative PEM study found no difference in the incidence of jaundice (4). Although this does not exclude the estolate as an occasional cause of jaundice, there was certainly no evidence that it is a relatively more common cause. In another study, we looked at about 16,000 patients treated with emepronium bromide, which was associated with occasional reports of esophagitis. Approximately 450 doctors reported that patients had indeed experienced some swallowing difficulty after taking the tablets; these positive replies were so numerous that we were obligated to investigate the matter further using a four-page questionnaire. The secondary enquiry found that only a handful of patients had severe esophagitis and only one life had been threatened.

COMPARATIVE STUDIES OF NSAIDS

The value of PEM has been well illustrated by our studies of seven NSAIDs. Benoxaprofen was associated with a large number of reports of skin rashes, almost all due to photosensitivity. The possibility that photosensitivity might persist long after the drug had been withdrawn prompted us to conduct a special experiment three or four years later. We were also interested in determining the completeness of reporting to the CSM. We discovered, on following up more than 900 reports received by the DSRU, that at least one-third of these cases had also been reported to the CSM. We were able to show that reporting to the CSM had not been influenced significantly by the "Oraflex"-jaundice publicity. This suggested that we might need to modify our view that adverse reactions are grossly under-reported, by the voluntary methods. It is quite likely that many minor adverse reactions are under-reported but when the side effect is serious the reports to the CSM may be more complete than has been thought.

We analyzed indomethacin administered in the sophisticated delivery system known as "Osmosin," which releases the drug progressively as the capsule passes through the gut and thereby minimizes gastric intolerance. We discovered to our surprise that the rate for reports of gastritis or dyspepsia with this product was considerably greater than with four other products studied earlier (benoxaprofen, fenbufen, zomepirac, and piroxicam). However, when the drug was removed from the market, patients who had received it still experienced a much higher rate of dyspepsia and gastritis. When we ranked the drugs according to the frequency with which patients experienced this side effect, we found that the rate during treatment was directly proportional to the rate following treatment. The rates for indomethacin during and after treatment were the highest and those for piroxicam were the lowest. Our tentative conclusion was that, whenever a company promotes an NSAID as being less liable to produce certain side effects, doctors will tend to prescribe it for those patients who are most likely to develop those same side effects. One important consequence is that doctors will then report relatively more events with the seemingly less toxic drug. This has led us to the general conclusion that if you make something safer, people will take greater risks with it and thus cancel out the advantage (5).

When we came to look at the more serious side effects of NSAIDs, notably the complications of peptic ulceration, we failed to find any difference among the seven drugs in the frequency of gastrointestinal hemorrhage or perforation. Nor did we find any important differences between the rates for these complications during and after treatment. We have to accept, of course, that many patients who stopped treatment with one NSAID would have been switched to another.

POST-MARKETING SURVEILLANCE AND POST-MARKETING CLINICAL TRIALS

An important distinction needs to be made between post-marketing surveillance and post-marketing clinical trials. Post-marketing surveillance is conducted under "real life" conditions in which events are ascertained in patients for whom a therapeutic decision has already been made. The surveillance procedure must not influence the choice of treatment. In post-marketing clinical trials, on the other hand, a patient's treatment is deliberately changed and is followed up prospectively. In these circumstances a patient must be a fully informed volunteer.

In the United Kingdom, Intercontinental Medical Statistics Limited (IMS) recently established a Post-marketing Surveillance Unit which is engaged in what seem to be post-marketing clinical trials rather than PMS. Their procedure is quite different from ours. They write to physicians encouraging them to take part in a "PMS" study for which IMS offers financial remuneration. If the study were restricted to patients who had already commenced treatment one could argue that it was truly post-marketing surveillance. In practice, however, their approach encourages physicians to change patients' treatments and the study is therefore technically a promotional post-marketing clinical trial. This distinction is extremely important because the results of post-marketing clinical trials of this kind differ very significantly from those of real-life post-marketing surveillance. In the former, there may be a considerable element of selection. For example, doctors may avoid use of the new drugs in high-risk groups such as elderly patients, pregnant women, children, and so on.

We recently encountered an important example of this difference. We compared the results of a large post-marketing clinical trial of enalapril in approximately 11,700 patients, and a PEM study of more than 13,000 patients conducted by the DSRU. In the first, study patients were observed for only six weeks, and there were eight deaths. In the PEM study, which covered a year of observation, there were 1,098 deaths. Adjusting for the difference in duration of the studies, this rate was about 80 times greater than in the clinical trial. There were 152 reports of renal failure, of which 75 were fatal. No cases of renal failure had been reported in the clinical trial. Fortunately for enalapril, the CSM agreed to wait until we fully investigated the reports of renal failure and in particular the 75 deaths. After intensive study involving colleagues from the Post-Graduate Medical School in London, Sir Colin Dollery and Christopher Speirs, we were able to show that all but perhaps 10 of the fatal cases of renal failure could be accounted for by pre-existing renal disease. Even in the 10 deaths in which enalapril might have played a part, other factors such as excessive use of diuretics or hyperkalemia could well have precipitated the renal failure (6,7).

The large differences between these two studies can be accounted for almost entirely by selection. The company study was conducted in low-risk patients with middle to moderate hypertension. The PEM study reflected, very precisely, a widely varying range of patients receiving enalapril. Many were suffering from advanced congestive heart failure and a proportion had pre-existing renal disease. If the company made a mistake it was calling their study post-marketing surveillance when it was plainly a post-marketing clinical trial.

Another problem, which is causing us considerable concern, is the distortion of early prescribing practice by some company studies in which a small number of doctors are encouraged to prescribe for large numbers of patients. Recently, for example, we encountered a drug which was the subject of a company study where 5 percent of the doctors who prescribed it accounted for more than half the total U.K. market. In one extreme case a doctor had prescribed the drug for 235 patients during the six months following its introduction. This drug was licensed for use only for rheumatoid arthritis.

Sooner or later another unexpected incident like practolol is almost inevitable. Our best hope lies in its early detection and containment. The speed with which we identify a hazard depends upon the speed with which we can gather sufficient information about the largest possible number of patients. Competition for patients early in the market life of a new drug will inevitably fragment the available data base and lead to a failure to identify an unexpected hazard. We have already seen several examples where promotional studies conducted by drug companies or market research organizations have seriously delayed the progress of PEM. Guidelines for post-marketing surveillance in the United Kingdom insist that it should not be promotional. If this were true there would be no need for such studies to compete with the two national systems, PEM and the yellow card scheme. After these systems establish that a new drug has an acceptable level of safety, the companies should be able to continue their sales drive with greater confidence.

CONCLUSION

Despite a close working relationship with the government and the pharmaceutical industry, the DRSU's greatest asset is its independence from both. This has given it credibility and considerable influence, particularly in regulatory circles. Using the United Kingdom's unique ability to identify all patients who receive a particular drug, we can study its performance rapidly in large numbers of patients. The cost is quite modest; a one-year study of 10,000 patients, including follow-up of any who die or develop serious adverse reactions, costs on average $400,000. We have all been looking for inexpensive monitoring of health outcomes in the real world of clinical practice. I would like to think that, in Prescription-Event Monitoring, we have gone some way toward achieving that goal.

REFERENCES

1. Inman WHW. Detection and investigation of drug safety problems. In Gent M, Shigamatsu I (eds). Epidemiological Issues in Reported Drug-Induced Illnesses. Hamilton, Ontario: McMaster University Library Press, 1976.
2. Inman WHW, Weber JCP. In Inman WHW (ed). Monitoring for Drug Safety. Second edition. Lancaster, England: MTP Press, 1986:37.
3. Inman WHW, Rawson NSB, Wilton LV. Prescription-Event Monitoring. In Inman WHW (ed). Monitoring for Drug Safety. Second edition. Lancaster, England: MTP Press, 1986:213–235.
4. Inman WHW, Rawson NSB. Erythromycin estolate and jaundice. British Medical Journal 1983;286:1954–1955.
5. Inman WHW. Risks in medical intervention. In Cooper M. (ed). Risk: Man-Made Hazards to Man. Oxford: Oxford University Press, 1985.
6. Inman WHW, Rawson NSB, Wilton LV, Pearce GL, Speirs CL. Post-marketing surveillance of enalapril. I: Results of prescription-event monitoring. British Medical Journal 1988;297:826–829.
7. Speirs CJ, Dollery CT, Inman WHW, Rawson NSB, Wilton LV. Post-marketing surveillance of enalapril. II: Investigation of the potential role of enalapril in deaths with renal failure. British Medical Journal 1988;297:830–832.

7

The Role of Decision Analysis in the Translation of Research Findings into Clinical Practice

ALBERT G. MULLEY, JR.

The purpose of this paper is to consider the potential of decision analysis for improving the transfer of the fruits of clinical research into clinical practice, where health benefits can be realized. A narrow view of that potential might focus on the use of decision analysis to synthesize research findings in the context of existing evidence. Indeed, decision analysis has been used extensively to help define the clinical role of new drugs, devices, and procedures (1,2). Examples include drugs and procedures to treat coronary disease, devices to crush kidney stones or gallstones, immunoassays to detect disease or protect the blood supply, and devices that provide images of normal and diseased human anatomy. But if we consider these examples, or other new drugs, devices, or procedures on the horizon, it seems clear that the "demand-pull" of clinical practice is at least as powerful a force as the "innovation-push" of science and technology. Human problems translate into clinical problems and those clinical problems stimulate investigation. Intelligence must move between clinical investigation and clinical practice in both directions. Decision analysis can emphasize the interactive nature of this process and thereby improve both the efficiency of clinical investigation and the timely clinical application of new technologies.

DECISION ANALYSIS AT THE INTERFACE BETWEEN CLINICAL INVESTIGATION AND CLINICAL PRACTICE

Decision analysis can facilitate the interactive transfer of information between clinical investigation and clinical practice by assisting in three functions: (a) setting priorities and identifying clinically important parameters for

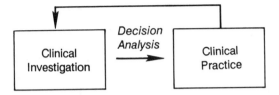

A Role for Decision Analysis

- Setting priorities and parameters for clinical investigation

- Synthesizing, interpreting, disseminating results of clinical investigation

- Distinguishing between matters of fact and value judgments . . . Implications for Agency

FIGURE 7.1 The role of decision analysis at the interface between clinical investigation and clinical practice.

clinical investigation; (b) synthesizing, interpreting, and disseminating the results of clinical investigation; and (c) making important distinctions between matters of fact—the evidence produced by clinical investigation—and the value judgments inherent in decisions about use of new drugs, devices, and technologies. This last function draws attention to agency and perspective: the clinician's role as rational agent for patients, the investigator or developer's responsibility to the public and prospective patients, and government officials' responsibility to protect the public welfare (see Figure 7.1). To understand how decision analysis can be helpful with these functions, its strengths and limitations must be understood.

WHAT DECISION ANALYSIS IS

Decision analysis is a systematic approach to decisions that have to be made in the face of uncertainty (3,4,5). It is systematic for three reasons. It requires an explicit formulation of the problem, including alternative choices that are available to the decision maker and important specific outcomes. This formulation is often represented by a figure called a decision tree. Second, it requires the explicit quantitative representation of uncertainty in the form of probabilities. Third, it requires the explicit quantitative representation of preferences in the form of utilities.

Decision analysis is potentially prescriptive. If one is willing to assign probabilities to all uncertain events and utilities to all outcomes, and accept assumptions inherent in the expected utility model, decision analysis can prescribe the course of action that should be followed. For some, this prescriptive intent of decision analysis is cause for skepticism, often because it is misunderstood.

The very simple decision tree represented by Figure 7.2 illustrates the explicit nature of decision analysis and the expected utility model. In this case, just two options are available to the decision maker. If the choice is alternative 1, the outcome is uncertain. There is a chance that the outcome will be "healthy," but there is also a chance that the outcome will be state j. If alternative 2 is chosen, the decision maker can be certain that the outcome will be state i.

This simple model captures the essence of the clinical decision involving a patient whose condition, state i, could either be cured or made worse (state j) by a particular intervention (alternative 1). The decision analyst would insist on an explicit, precise estimate of the probability of cure and the complementary probability of harm. Preferences for states i and j, relative to being healthy, would be expressed quantitatively as utilities. The sum of the utilities of "healthy" and state j, weighted by their respective probabilities, would be the expected utility or benefit of alternative 1. The expected benefit of alternative 1 minus that of alternative 2 (in this case, simply 1 multiplied by the utility of state i), would be the net expected benefit. If it were positive, alternative 1 would be advised; if negative, alternative 2 would be advised. As noted, willingness to make a decision based on the expected value of an alternative course of action depends on acceptance of the expected utility model.

The results of decision analyses often seem overly precise. After all, probability estimates may be highly uncertain and preferences may vary greatly among different raters and across time. But if explicit formulation of problems and representation of uncertainty and preferences is the first virtue of the

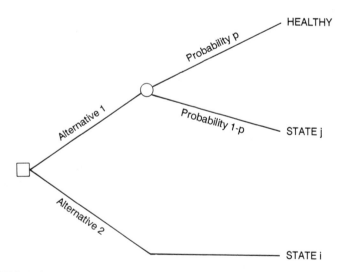

FIGURE 7.2 A simple decision tree. Square nodes represent decision points; round nodes represent chance events.

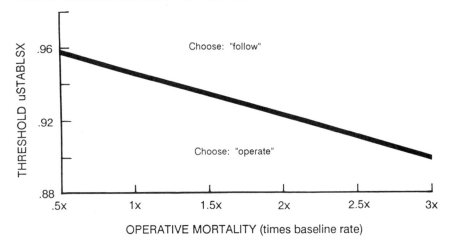

FIGURE 7.3 A two-way sensitivity analysis that displays results of a decision analysis for men with symptoms of benign prostatic hyperplasia who are considering TURP. The decision depends on operative mortality and utility associated with the baseline symptom state. SOURCE: Barry MJ, Mulley AG, Fowler FJ, Wennberg JE. Watchful waiting versus immediate transurethral resection for symptomatic prostatism: The importance of patients' preferences. Journal of the American Medical Association 1988;259:3010-3017.

method, flexibility is the second. Problem formulation can be altered, and probabilities or utilities can be varied across a plausible range, to estimate the sensitivity of the result, which is the net expected benefit of the preferred option. Specific "threshold" values can be identified for probabilities (e.g., of state j) or utilities (e.g., of state i) at which the net expected benefit changes from positive to negative, and the preferred option thereby changes.

Figure 7.3 is an example of a two-way sensitivity analysis drawn from a detailed model of the decision to perform transurethral resection of the prostate (TURP). This procedure is used to improve quality of life that has been diminished by the symptoms of prostatism; note that life with these symptoms is analogous to state i in our simple model (6). The figure depicts the threshold utility for the symptom state that would make the expected utility of surgery just equal to the expected utility of "watchful waiting" for a range of operative mortality rates. It is this flexibility of decision analysis that gives it the potential to help set priorities for clinical investigation and effectively transfer research findings to clinical practice.

THE LIMITATIONS OF DECISION ANALYSIS: WHAT IT IS NOT

Decision analysis is a powerful method when used appropriately, but appropriate use requires recognition of some important limitations. Decision analysis is not a substitute for knowledge. The method does nothing to reduce uncertainty faced by the decision maker. Rather, it forces an untangling of multiple uncertainties and helps identify those that most affect the choice.

In this context it is worth considering the kinds of uncertainty that can be represented by probabilities in a decision analytic model (7). First, there is the personal uncertainty that exists when a decision maker is unaware of information that others have. Using a probability to represent one's strength of belief under these circumstances may be less appropriate than education, depending on the availability of the information and the urgency of the decision. Second, there is the collective uncertainty of the professional community. This may reflect the unfinished business of clinical research that has not been performed, or more difficult questions that are less amenable to investigation. In either case, if decisions must be made now, there is no good alternative to the most informed opinion. The decision analyst would express that opinion in the form of a subjective probability estimate. Finally, there is the stochastic uncertainty that always exists when dealing with biologic systems and human behavior. This element of chance will persist no matter how precisely we can estimate a probability based on past experience under similar circumstances.

Another problem is that decision analysis is not descriptive. To describe the analytic approach, which depends heavily on the expected utility model, is not to describe the way most people behave. There is, however, a very rich body of descriptive decision theory that provides an important, often unappreciated, complement to decision analysis (8,9). By identifying patterns in actual decision-making behavior, this theory can sensitize us to differences between the way we behave and the way we ought to behave if we subscribe to the axioms of rational choice that form the basis for decision analysis. The choice remains with the decision maker. Decision analysis is not necessarily prescriptive.

SETTING PRIORITIES AND PARAMETERS FOR CLINICAL INVESTIGATION

The explicit formulation of a decision problem and the use of probabilities to represent uncertainty can prevent errors of intuition in anticipating the impact of a new drug, device, or procedure. However, the principal role of decision analysis in setting priorities and parameters for clinical investigation is in forcing an orientation to health outcomes and the values associated with them. The formulation of a decision analytic model makes us consider which health outcomes are important, and how important they are relative to one another.

Decision analysis also facilitates consideration of the potential marginal benefit of a new intervention by forcing comparisons with other alternatives or "fallback positions." In the example already presented, the effect of TURP on health outcome must be compared with the effect of the alternative, watchful waiting. It is the comparison that gives us the estimate of net expected benefit. As obvious as this may seem, there are countless examples where insufficient attention is paid to the fallback position, both in establishing criteria for appropriate use of existing technologies and in embarking on clinical investigation to estimate the potential contribution of new technologies.

The requirement for explicit formulations and the orientation toward outcome and value provide a real advantage for those who would establish priorities and set parameters for clinical investigation. Clinical research tends to focus on the efficacy of a particular drug or procedure, or on the sensitivity and specificity of a diagnostic test. Often it does not consider the string of uncertainties and choices that precede or follow an action and that provide the links between the initial choice among alternatives and the valued outcomes. We well know that mistakes with profound implications are made when such a succession of choices, contingent events, and conditional probabilities are considered intuitively rather than systematically (10).

The systematic approach can be used to set parameters for clinical research. For example, the design of a clinical trial can establish the clinically important difference in efficacy, used with alpha and beta errors to calculate sample size, by using a sensitivity analysis that varies relative efficacy of the new intervention as opposed to the available alternatives. Such an approach may be even more valuable when establishing parameters for performance of diagnostic tests rather than therapeutic interventions. The following example illustrates this point.

Currently, there is substantial excitement and some controversy about the development of a new serologic assay that could protect the blood supply against the transmission of non-A non-B hepatitis. Yet tests that would offer some protection have been available for many years. Alanine aminotransferase (ALT) testing has not been implemented because, with a sensitivity of only 30 percent and a specificity of 92 percent (i.e., 8 percent of donated blood would have to be discarded because of false-positive results), it did not seem worth the cost. However, when one considers the health and cost implications of non-A non-B hepatitis, it becomes apparent that there is a broad range of sensitivity-specificity pairs for which ALT testing would not only prevent morbidity and mortality but also save health care dollars (11). The estimated sensitivity and specificity of ALT testing fall well within this range (see Figure 7.4).

The term "fallback position," used earlier, is adapted from Phelps and Muslin (12), who have used a similar approach to establish priorities for the evaluation of magnetic resonance imaging (MRI). They perform decision analyses to put the information that MRI might provide in a particular clinical situation in an outcome-oriented context. They first ask whether MRI would make a positive contribution to health outcome if it were perfectly sensitive and specific. In other words, is knowing the diagnosis for the condition under consideration at a particular point in its course going to make a difference? If that hurdle is passed, how much better does MRI have to be than a less costly fallback test (or, in the case of tests other than MRI that involve risk of morbidity, a less

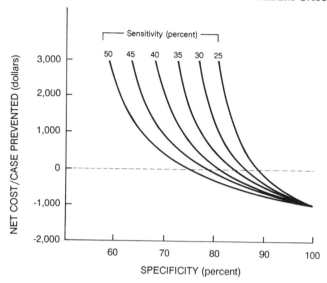

FIGURE 7.4 The net cost per case of non-A non-B hepatitis prevented by use of a screening test as it varies with the sensitivity and specificity of the test. SOURCE: Silverstein MD, Mulley AG, Dienstag JL. Should donor blood be screened for elevated alanine aminotransferase levels? A cost-effectiveness analysis. Journal of the American Medical Association 1984;252:2839-2845.

risky test) to justify its use? Phelps and Muslin answer the question with a receiver operating characteristic curve that displays a "challenge region" for MRI (see Figure 7.5). Again, the result is more targeted clinical investigation with clear and explicit definition of the "clinically important difference."

SYNTHESIZING, INTERPRETING, AND DISSEMINATING RESULTS OF CLINICAL RESEARCH

The characteristics of decision analysis that make it valuable for setting priorities and parameters are useful in bringing the results of research to clinical practice. Sensitivity and threshold analyses can be used to consider the limits to external validity of a clinical study more explicitly and systematically. The efficacy or complication rates seen in the highly selected populations that participate in clinical trials can be varied across a wide range to determine the impact of either decreased effectiveness or greater risk on overall outcome. The previously mentioned TURP analysis is an example (see Figure 7.3).

The same approach has been used to define levels of risk that warrant preventive interventions. Figure 7.6 summarizes the results of an analysis performed to determine indications for vaccination against hepatitis B, based primarily on cost considerations (13). The figure displays estimates of the cost per prevented case of hepatitis when the vaccine is used in populations facing dif-

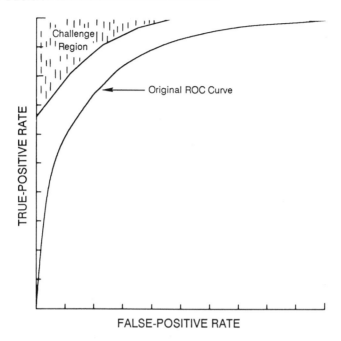

FIGURE 7.5 Use of receiver operating characteristic (ROC) curves to define the challenge region for a new diagnostic test. The original ROC curve displays the performance characteristics of an available test. The challenge region displays the range of improved performance characteristics that would justify a more costly or risky alternative. SOURCE: Phelps CE, Muslin AI. Focusing technology assessment using medical decision theory. Medical Decision Making 1988;8:279-289.

ferent attack rates. Costs below zero indicate that the vaccine would actually save money. This analysis is a good example of the iterative, bidirectional process that decision analysis can facilitate; it puts the results of the randomized trial in context, while focusing additional research efforts aimed at identifying hepatitis risk for different populations.

DISTINCTIONS BETWEEN MATTERS OF FACT, OR EVIDENCE, AND VALUE JUDGMENTS

Clinical research generally addresses questions that are represented by probabilities in a decision analysis. These are matters of evidence or fact. When translating these results to clinical practice, it is important to recognize the variability of different patients' utilities (14). For example, the vertical axis in Figure 7.3 may be related indirectly to many objective measures of symptom severity for men with prostate disease. That analysis further demonstrated that

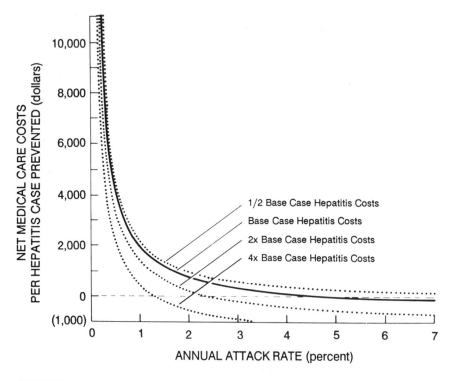

FIGURE 7.6 Net medical care costs per case of hepatitis prevented by vaccination of susceptible populations with different annual attack rates. SOURCE: Mulley AG, Silverstein MD, Dienstag JL. Indications for use of hepatitis B vaccine, based on cost-effectiveness analysis. New England Journal of Medicine 1982;307:644-652.

the range of values justifying surgery on the basis of baseline symptoms and operative mortality is increasingly constrained as patients' dislike of the potential loss of sexual function increases (6).

PRIORITIES FOR DECISION ANALYSTS

Decision analysis is underused at the interface between clinical research and clinical practice. Those who would like to see its use increase should address a number of priorities. First, there must be more and better examples of iterative work involving clinical investigation, decision analysis, and clinical practice. Too often decision analysts do their work and leave it at that. Too often clinical investigators pay no attention. There needs to be more collaborative work. Second, the field needs better integration of prescriptive decision theory (i.e., decision analysis) and descriptive decision theory. Prospect theory, regret theory, and other formulations of usual deviations from the expected utility model promote understanding of the analytic strengths of the prescriptive method and its problems. Third, we need better measurements of patients' preferences (14). Methods borrowed from economists and psychometricians may suffice for the scaling task. But we need a clinical theory based on the variability of preferences among persons and across time. Finally, decision theorists should pay more attention to the single-actor perspective of both prescriptive and descriptive decision theory. Most clinical decisions are made by parties who share unequally in information, experience, ability to make the relevant value judgments, and decision-making responsibility. Ideally, as decision analysis progresses in these directions it will become even more valuable at the interface between clinical investigation and clinical practice.

REFERENCES

1. Kassirer JP, Moskowitz AJ, Lau K, Pauker SG. Decision analysis: A progress report. Annals of Internal Medicine 1987;106:275–291.
2. Pauker SG, Kassirer JP. Decision analysis. New England Journal of Medicine 1987;316:250–257.
3. Raiffa H. Decision Analysis: Introductory Lectures on Choice Under Uncertainty. Reading, Mass.: Addison-Wesley, 1968.
4. Weinstein MC, Fineberg HV. Clinical Decision Analysis. Philadelphia: W. B. Saunders, 1980.
5. Sox HC Jr, Blatt MA, Higgins MC, Marton KI. Medical Decision Making. Boston: Butterworth, 1988.
6. Barry MJ, Mulley AG, Fowler FJ, Wennberg JE. Watchful waiting versus immediate transurethral resection for symptomatic prostatism: The importance of patients' preferences. Journal of the American Medical Association 1988;259:3010–3017.
7. Mulley AG. Medical decision making and practice variation. In Andersen TF, Mooney G (eds). The Challenges of Medical Practice Variation. London, U.K.: Macmillan, in press.
8. Kahneman D, Slovic P, Tversky A (eds). Judgement Under Uncertainty : Heuristics and Biases. Cambridge, U.K.: Cambridge University Press, 1982.
9. Elstein AS. Clinical judgment: Psychological research and medical practice. Science 1976;194:696–700.
10. Eddy DM, Billings J. The quality of medical evidence: Implications for quality of health care. Health Affairs 1988;7:19–32.
11. Silverstein MD, Mulley AG, Dienstag JL. Should donor blood be screened for elevated alanine aminotransferase levels? A cost-effectiveness analysis. Journal of the American Medical Association 1984;252:2839–2845.
12. Phelps CE, Muslin AI. Focusing technology assessment using medical decision theory. Medical Decision Making 1988;8:279–289.
13. Mulley AG, Silverstein MD, Dienstag JL. Indications for use of hepatitis B vaccine, based on cost-effectiveness analysis. New England Journal of Medicine 1982;307:644–652.
14. Mulley, AG. Assessing patients' utilities: Can the ends justify the means? Medical Care 1989;27:S269–S281.

8

Meta-Analysis: A Quantitative Approach to Research Integration*

STEPHEN B. THACKER

The goal of an integrative literature review is to summarize the accumulated knowledge concerning a field of interest and to highlight important issues that researchers have left unresolved (1). Traditionally, the medical literature has been integrated in the narrative form. An expert in a field will review studies, decide which are relevant, and highlight his or her findings, both in terms of results and, to a lesser degree, methodology. Topics for further research may also be proposed. Such narrative reviews have two basic weaknesses (2,3). First, no systematic approach is prescribed to obtain primary data or to integrate findings; rather, the subjective judgment of the reviewer is used. As a result, no explicit standards exist to assess the quality of a review. Second, the narrative reviewer does not synthesize data quantitatively across literature. Consequently, as the number of studies in any discipline increases, so does the probability that erroneous conclusions will be reached in a narrative review (4).

Scientific research is founded on integration and replication of results; with the possible exception of a new discovery, a single study rarely makes a dramatic contribution to the advancement of knowledge (5). In this article I summarize the constraints on reviewers of the medical literature and review alternative methods for synthesizing scientific studies. In particular, I examine meta-analysis, a quantitative method to combine data, and illustrate with a clinical example its application to the medical literature. Then, I describe the strengths and weakness of meta-analysis and approaches to its evaluation. Finally, I discuss

---

*This paper was previously published in The Journal of the American Medical Association 1988;259:1685-1689.

current research issues related to meta-analysis and highlight future research directions.

CONSTRAINTS ON LITERATURE REVIEW

The limitations of any approach to literature review can be summarized as follows (6): (a) sampling bias due to reporting and publication policies; (b) the absence in published studies of specific data desired for review; (c) biased exclusion of studies by the investigator; (d) the uneven quality of the primary data; and (e) biased outcome interpretation. These concerns are applicable to any form of literature review.

Two types of bias in the published literature must concern a reviewer. First, because authors and journal editors tend to report statistically significant findings, a review limited to published studies will tend to overestimate the effect size. In a survey, for example, 58 investigators indicated that they had conducted 921 randomized controlled trials, and that 96 (21.3 percent) were unpublished. Positive randomized controlled trials were significantly more likely to be published than negative trials (77 percent versus 42 percent, P < .001) (7). At the same time, one should not uncritically assume that methods are better in published studies, as the quality of published papers varies dramatically (8). Second, another form of publication bias, the confirmatory bias, tends to emphasize and believe experiences that support one's views and to ignore or discredit those that do not. Results of a study of 75 journal reviewers asked to referee identical experimental procedures showed poor interrater agreement and a bias against results contrary to their theoretical perspective (9). Consequently, new or unpopular data tend also to be underreported in the published literature.

Data available from primary research studies may be inadequate for the literature reviewer. The reviewer is often confronted with selective reporting of primary findings, incorrect primary data analysis, and inadequate descriptions of original studies (10). In a study of psychotherapy outcomes, for example, an effect could not be calculated in 26 percent of studies because of missing data, a number comparable with previous reports (11).

In addition to identifying studies, the investigator must decide which reports to include in a review (3). One option is to use all available data and thereby maximize the representativeness of the conclusions. Using this approach, however, one will decrease the statistical validity of the data synthesis by including less rigorous studies. Exclusion of studies for methodological reasons, on the other hand, will increase the statistical validity but will decrease the size of the overall pool of data and may sacrifice the ability to generalize from the results.

Variable data quality is probably the most critical limitation for the reviewer. The effect of data quality was seen in a study of quality of life outcomes following coronary bypass graft surgery, when investigators found the estimates of benefit to be 15 percent less in randomized controlled trials than in trials using matching (12). Similarly, results of studies in medical care tend to show decreasing odds ratios with increased rigor of studies (8), although in one large study of psychotherapy, the effect was found to increase with increasing rigor (11). In quantitative reviews, statistical methods, including stratified analyses and multivariate methods, can be used to measure the impact on the results of varying quality in studies (8,13,14).

Although these constraints have been recognized previously, the more recent efforts to address concerns about research integration have stimulated new efforts to deal with them.

QUANTITATIVE APPROACHES TO SUMMARIZING ACROSS STUDIES

During the past several years, there have been several different approaches developed to summarize quantitatively data found in different studies of the same or similar research problems. The simplest approach to the quantitative integration of research is vote counting. With this approach, results of studies under consideration are classified into three categories: (a) statistically significant in one direction, (b) statistically significant in the opposite direction, or (c) no statistically significant difference. Then, the category receiving the most votes is judged to approximate truth (15). Although simple to use, voting methods do not take into account the magnitude of effect or sample size. In addition, this approach does not address the aforementioned problems inherent in traditional reviews, such as inadequate study methodology and uneven data quality.

In 1971, Light and Smith (15) proposed an alternative to voting methods that takes advantage of natural aggregations, or clusters, in the population. In this approach, one studies a problem in various clusters, such as neighborhoods or classrooms, and searches for explanations for differences among clusters. If these differences are explainable, the data can be combined and statistical variability can be described.

A third method for combining literature is pooling, a method by which data from multiple studies of a single topic, such as β-blockade after myocardial infarction, are combined in a single analysis (16). This method is limited by the availability of raw data; the variation in study methods, populations, and outcomes under study; and statistical considerations (17,18).

In a 1976 study of the efficacy of psychotherapy, Glass (19) coined the term meta-analysis, "the statistical analysis of a large collection of results from individual literature, for the purpose of integrating the findings." Alternatively, meta-analysis can be defined as any systematic method that uses statistical analyses for combining data from independent studies to obtain a numerical estimate of the overall effect of a particular procedure or variable on a defined outcome (20).

While there have been several approaches to meta-analysis, the steps can be defined generally as (a) defining the problem and criteria for admission of studies, (b) locating research studies, (c) classifying and coding study characteristics, (d) quantitatively measuring study characteristics on a common scale, (e) aggregating study findings and relating findings to study characteristics (analysis and interpretation), and (f) reporting the results (21,22).

Problem formulation includes the explicit definition of both outcomes and potentially confounding variables. Carefully done, this step enables the investigator to focus on the relevant measures in the studies under consideration and to specify relevant methods to classify and code study characteristics.

The literature search includes a systematic approach to locating studies (1). First, one obtains information from the so-called invisible college, i.e., the informal exchange of information among colleagues in a particular discipline. Second, one searches indexes (e.g., Index Medicus and the Social Science Citation Index), abstracting services (e.g., International Pharmaceutical Abstracts), and computerized searches (e.g., MEDLINE and TOXLINE) to obtain research articles and sources of both published and unpublished data. Third, references in available studies identify further sources. The retrieval from academic, private, and government researchers of unreferenced reports, the so-called fugitive literature, as well as unpublished data, further minimizes selective reporting and publication biases.

Several methods are used to measure the results across studies (3,23). The most commonly used measure in the social sciences is the effect size, an index of both the direction and magnitude of the effect of a procedure under study (19). Glass and his colleagues (24) developed this method when assessing the efficacy of psychotherapy on the basis of data from controlled studies. One estimate of effect size for quantitative data is the difference between two group means divided by the control group SD: $(X_t - X_c)/S_c$, where X_t is the mean of the experimental or exposed group, X_c is the mean of the control or unexposed group, and S_c is the SD of the control group. Effect size expresses differences in SD units so that, for example, if a study has an effect size of 0.2 SD units, the overall effect size is half that of another study that has an effect size of 0.4 SD units. The appropriate measure of effect across literature will vary according both to the nature of the problem being assessed and to the availability of published data (7,25). Pooling of data from controlled clinical trials, for example, has been more widely used in the medical literature (16,26).

Effect size for proportions has been calculated in cohort literature as either a difference, $P_t - P_c$, or as a ratio, P_t/P_c (3). The latter has the advantage of considering the change relative to the control percentage and, in epidemiologic studies, is equivalent analytically to the concept of the risk ratio.

Whatever combination statistic is used, a systematic quantitative procedure to accumulate results across studies should include the following (27): (a) summary descriptive statistics across studies and the averaging of those statistics; (b) calculation of the variance of a statistic across studies (i.e., tests for heterogeneity); (c) correction of the variance by subtracting sampling error; (d) correction in the mean and variance for study artifacts other than sampling, such as measurement error; and (e) comparison of the corrected SD to the mean to assess the size of the potential variation across studies. A growing literature on statistical methods deals with problems in calculating effect size or significance testing as it relates to meta-analysis (28,29).

BENEFITS OF META-ANALYSIS

Meta-analysis forces systematic thought about methods, outcomes, categorizations, populations, and interventions as one accumulates evidence. In addition, it offers a mechanism for estimating the magnitude of effect in terms of a statistically significant effect size or pooled odds ratio. Furthermore, the combination of data from several studies increases generalizability and potentially increases statistical power, thus enabling one to assess more completely the impact of a procedure or variable (30). Quantitative measures across studies can also give insight into the nature of relationships among variables and provide a mechanism for detecting and exploring apparent contradictions in results. Finally, users of meta-analysis have expressed the hope that this systematic approach would be less subjective and would decrease investigator bias.

APPLICATIONS OF META-ANALYSIS IN HEALTH

Interest in clinical applications of meta-analysis has risen dramatically in recent years (31,32). An increasing number of attempts have been made to use meta-analysis outside of mental health or educational settings, including such other settings as chemotherapy in breast cancer (33), patient education interventions in clinical medicine (34), spinal manipulation (35), the effects of exercise on serum lipid levels (36), and duodenal ulcer therapy (37). There has also been discussion of the potential applications of meta-analysis to public health (38). An interesting application of meta-analysis was an effort to quantify the impact on survival and safety of a wide range of surgical and anesthetic innovations (39). More typical are efforts to draw conclusions from data pooled from a limited number of studies, usually controlled clinical trials (26,40-47). Pooling techniques have also been applied to data from non-randomized studies in attempts to address incompletely studied problems and to increase representativeness (25,48,49).

A CASE STUDY: ELECTRONIC FETAL MONITORING

In a 1979 review of the efficacy and safety of intrapartum electronic fetal monitoring, Banta and Thacker (50) set out to assess the evidence for the efficacy and safety of the routine use of electronic fetal monitoring. The independent variable was defined as the clinical application of all forms of electronic fetal monitoring to both high- and low-risk pregnant women; the outcomes measured were various measures of maternal and fetal morbidity and mortality, as well as the occurrence of cesarean delivery. Cost issues were also addressed.

A literature search began with the exchange of information with colleagues in obstetrics, pediatrics, epidemiology, technology assessment, and economics. References to published research articles were obtained from MEDLINE and Index Medicus and supplemented with references in articles under review. Efforts were also made to obtain unpublished reports and professional meeting abstracts. Although this review was systematic and extensive and comparable evidence from studies was sought, a quantitative analysis across studies was limited to descriptive statistics.

A 1987 meta-analysis of this same issue focused on evidence from randomized controlled trials and the previous literature search supplemented with information from the Oxford Data Base of Perinatal Trials and from direct correspondence with individual investigators (51). Variables were codified and, where possible, made comparable. For example, published measures of the Apgar score varied in timing (at 1, 2, and 5 minutes) and classification (abnormal was defined variably to include or exclude a score of 7); authors were asked to provide one-minute Apgar scores where a normal score included 7.

The primary data were then organized into descriptive tables that listed study results for specific outcomes, such as low Apgar score, perinatal mortality, and cesarean delivery, as well as for measures of diagnostic precision, such as sensitivity, specificity, and predictive value (see Table 8.1) (50). The findings of the randomized controlled trials were evaluated for comparability and then pooled (see Table 8.2), and the pooled analyses were stratified by data quality (51). The results of the pooled analyses were then reported, conclusions were drawn, and recommendations were made.

TABLE 8.1 Accuracy of electronic fetal monitoring using Apgar score as measure of outcome[a]

Investigator, year	Number of Patients	PPV	NPV	Sensitivity, %	Specificity,%
Bissonnette (69), 1975	714	80	94	57	82
Gabert and Stenchever (70), 1973	749	66	91	84	80
Schifrin and Dame (71), 1972	307	43	93	54	90
Saldana et al. (72), 1976	620	23	86	71	44
Tipton and Shelley (73), 1971	100	81	93	82	93

[a]Abnormality defined as one-minute Apgar score < 7 (except Gabert—one-minute Apgar score < 6).
PPV, positive predictive value; NPV, negative predictive value.

TABLE 8.2 Pooled data from six controlled trials assessing efficacy of routine electronic fetal monitoring in labor

	Pooled Odds Ratio	95% Confidence Interval	Test for Heterogeneity[a]
Apgar score < 7	1.07	0.88 – 1.30	$\chi^2_6 = 1.28$
Apgar score < 4	0.87	0.56 – 1.30	$\chi^2_5 = 1.84$
Neonatal seizures	0.39	0.14 – 1.08	$\chi^2_6 = 3.75$
NICU admissions	1.01	0.84 – 1.22	$\chi^2_6 = 12.15$
Perinatal deaths	1.73	0.53 – 5.64	$\chi^2_6 = 5.51$

[a]All tests were not significant. The subscript numbers refer to degrees of freedom.
NICU, neonatal intensive care unit.

The 1979 study concluded that the data did not support the routine use of electronic fetal monitoring and recommended additional randomized controlled trials and limitation of electronic fetal monitoring to high-risk pregnancies (50). The 1987 report included randomized controlled trials already cited in the original study and three additional randomized controlled trials (seven randomized controlled trials from five countries). No known clinical trials were excluded from this report although the largest trial (52), which included more subjects than the other six in combination, was analyzed separately and compared with the pooled results of the others.

Analyses of different subsets of these studies based on differences in design (e.g., use of fetal scalp blood in sampling) and study quality found minor variations in results, but no changes in the basic findings. In both reports the pooled cesarean delivery rate was twofold higher in the group with electronic fetal monitoring. Data from the randomized controlled trial that scored highest in an assessment of the quality of study design and implementation, however, indicated that electronic fetal monitoring combined with fetal scalp blood sampling could be used to identify infants at risk of neonatal seizures (52). That study had been suggested by pooled analyses of earlier randomized controlled trials (53). While both of these reports illustrate the advantages of the systematic and comprehensive approach to a literature review, the meta-analytic methods used in the 1987 report illustrate both increased statistical power derived from data pooling and increased information found from stratification of studies. Subsequently available trials reported results consistent with that meta-analysis (54,55).

CRITICISMS OF META-ANALYSIS

When meta-analysis was introduced in the psychology literature, it did not meet with universal acceptance. It was variously described as "an exercise in mega-silliness" and "an abuse of research integration" (56,57). In addition to the constraints listed above related to literature review, the meta-analyst is confronted with additional challenges in an effort to synthesize data quantitatively across studies.

Statistical significance testing that is familiar to most clinicians is based on an assumption that data are selected randomly from a well-specified population. Non-random selection of studies and multiple tests of the same data, either through repeated publication of partial or entire data sets or through use of more than one outcome for each person, are two ways that this assumption is violated. Nevertheless, standard parametric statistics have been considered to be sufficiently robust to be usable in meta-analyses (58).

The current use of parametric statistical methods for meta-analysis requires additional theoretical study (29). Other methodological issues of concern to meta-analysts include bias (59), variability between studies (60), and the development of models to measure variability across studies (61). Additional statistical research should include study of the impact of outliers on the meta-analysis and the potential insight that they could provide into a research question (28). Statistically valid methods to combine data across studies of varying quality and design, including data from case-control studies, will enable meta-analysts to maximize the value of their data syntheses (48).

One serious concern about quantitative reviews of the literature is that although meta-analysis is more explicit, it may be no more objective than a narrative review (62). Both critics and advocates of meta-analysis are concerned that an unwarranted sense of scientific validity, rather than true understanding, may result from quantification (63,64). In other words, sophisticated statistics will not improve poor data but could lead to an unwarranted comfort with one's conclusions (65).

EVALUATION OF META-ANALYSIS

The evaluation of a literature review, like its conduct, should be systematic and quantitative. Evaluation criteria for meta-analysis include the need for the following: (a) clear identification of the problems under study; (b) active effort to include all available studies; (c) assessment of publication bias; (d) identification of data used; (e) selection and coding based on theoretical framework, not convenience; (f) detailed documentation of coding; (g) use of multiple raters to assess coding, including assessment of interrater reliability; (h) assessment of comparability of the cases, controls, and circumstances in the studies analyzed; (i) consideration of alternative explanations in the discussion; (j) relation of study characteristics to problems under review; (k) careful limitation of generalization to the domain of the literature review; (l) reporting in enough detail to enable replication by a reviewer; and (m) guidelines for future research (3,66).

COMMENT

Meta-analysis is an attempt to improve traditional methods of narrative review by systematically aggregating information and quantifying its impact. Meta-analysis was introduced to address the problem of synthesizing the large quantity of information on a particular subject, a problem that has been exacerbated by the large volume of published research in the past 20 years. It is viewed, however, only as a step in the process of developing better tools to quantify information across studies. It should neither be considered the final word in quantitative reviewing nor be dropped in haste because of the problems and criticisms discussed above. Certainly, benefits are to be obtained from systematic and rigorous review of available information, including increases in power and generalizability, better understanding of complex issues, identification of correlations among variables, and identification of gaps to be addressed by appropriate research.

When criticizing meta-analysis, one must distinguish between those problems that are inherent in any literature review and those that are specifically a problem with meta-analysis. For example, data quality, sampling bias, and data retrieval are limitations inherent in any literature review. Similarly, while outcome interpretation may be affected by the various styles of summarizing research findings, biases are not limited to the meta-analyst. On the other hand, one must be wary of inappropriate weight being given to a procedure just because it is quantitative, particularly when used by those who do not understand the limitations of the statistical methods utilized. Finally, critics should empirically test the impact of their criticisms so as to take meta-analysis or its alternative methods of quantitative summarization of research to the next level of usefulness.

It has been suggested that investigators should combine quantitative and qualitative review data to enable practitioners to apply results to individual patients or program problems (67). In this way, researchers can investigate issues that are important but difficult to quantify. Nonquantitative information, such as expert opinion and anecdotal evidence, does have a significant impact on policy. Finally, one must be concerned that although even the best meta-analysis may represent all available trials and relevant studies, it may not represent clinical practice because of the nature of how and where research is conducted (63).

Several things can be done to assess meta-analysis and to improve methods of quantitative review. First, one can compare the results of meta-analysis with those of narrative reviews to identify differences in interpretation and conclusions. In one study where a statistical procedure for summarizing research findings was compared with narrative reviews, it was found that the statistical reviewer was more likely to support the hypothesis both in direction and magnitude, although the basic recommendations did not differ between groups (68). A second important area of research is in statistical methodology. Both theoretical research into the assumptions of alternative methods and empirical research testing of the accuracy and efficiency of these methods need to be undertaken. Third, methods to assess the quality of meta-analysis need to be tested and refined (66). Finally, in assessing meta-analysis, one must be careful to limit the extrapolation of conclusions to the field of study covered by the literature review. Although this is true of any cumulative review, the boundaries of the review must be carefully delineated and interpretation confined to those boundaries.

In summary, the systematic, quantitative review and organization of the cumulative experience in a subject matter is fundamental to good scientific practice. Meta-analysis is a methodology that warrants testing and empirical evaluation. This is similarly true of alternative approaches to synthesizing information. The need to use available information optimally cannot be avoided by the rational scientist. The particular framework of review—be it meta-analysis or some other approach—should be addressed as an important scientific endeavor. The importance of addressing this issue must be underscored in an era where scientific information is increasing exponentially and the potential for application of these findings is unprecedented.

REFERENCES

1. Cooper HM. Scientific guidelines for conducting integrative research reviews. Review of Educational Research 1982;52:291–302.
2. Jackson GB. Methods for integrative reviews. Review of Educational Research 1980;50:438–460.
3. Light RJ, Pillemer DB. Summing Up the Science of Reviewing Research. Cambridge, Mass.: Harvard University Press, 1984.
4. Levine RL, Hunter JE. Regression methodology: Correlation, meta-analysis, confidence intervals, and reliability. Journal of Leisure Research 1983;15:323–343.
5. Fiske DW. The meta-analytic revolution in outcome research. Journal of Consulting and Clinical Psychology 1983;51:65–70.
6. Hattie JA, Hansford BC. Meta-analysis: A reflection on problems. Australian Journal of Psychology 1984;36:239–254.
7. Chan SS, Sacks HS, Chalmers TC. The epidemiology of unpublished randomized control trials, abstracted. Clinical Research 1982;30:234A.
8. Chalmers TC, Smith H Jr, Blackburn B et al. A method for assessing the quality of a randomized control trial. Controlled Clinical Trials 1981;2:31–49.
9. Mahoney MJ. Publication prejudices: An experimental study of confirmatory bias in the peer review system. Cognitive Therapy and Research 1977;1:161–175.
10. Searles JS. A methodological and empirical critique of psychotherapy outcome meta-analysis. Behaviour Research and Therapy 1985;23:453–463.
11. Landman JT, Dawes RM. Psychotherapy outcome: Smith and Glass' conclusions stand up under scrutiny. American Psychologist 1982;37:504–516.
12. Wortman PM, Yeaton WH. Cumulating quality of life results in controlled trials of coronary artery bypass graft surgery. Controlled Clinical Trials 1985;6:289–305.
13. Chalmers TC, Celano P, Sacks HS et al. Bias in treatment assignment in controlled clinical trials. New England Journal of Medicine 1983;309:1358–1361.

14. Yeaton WH, Wortman PM. Evaluation issues in medical research synthesis. In Yeaton WH, Wortman PM (eds). Issues in Data Synthesis. San Francisco: Jossey-Bass Publications, 1984:43–56.

15. Light RJ, Smith PV. Accumulating evidence: Procedures for resolving contradictions among different research studies. Harvard Educational Review 1971;41:429–471.

16. Yusef S, Peto R, Lewis J et al. Beta blockade during and after myocardial infarction: An overview of the randomized trials. Progress in Cardiovascular Diseases 1985;27:335–371.

17. Einarson TR, McGhain WF, Bootman JL et al. Meta-analysis: Quantitative integration of independent research results. American Journal of Hospital Pharmacy 1985;42:1957–1964.

18. Bryant FB, Wortman PM. Methodological issues in the meta-analysis of quasi-experiments. In Yeaton WH, Wortman PM (eds). Issues in Data Synthesis. San Francisco: Jossey-Bass Publications, 1984:15–24.

19. Glass GV. Primary, secondary, and meta-analysis of research. Educational Researcher 1976;5:3–8.

20. Leviton LC, Cook TD. What differentiates meta-analysis from other forms of review? Journal of Personality 1981;49:231–236.

21. Ottenbacher KJ, Petersen P. Quantitative reviewing of medical literature: An approach to synthesizing research results in clinical procedures. Clinical Pediatrics 1983;28:423–427.

22. Curlette WL, Cannella KS. Going beyond the narrative summarization of research findings: The meta-analysis approach. Research in Nursing and Health 1985;8:293–301.

23. Rosenthal R. Combining results of independent studies. Psychological Bulletin 1978;85:185–193.

24. Glass GV, McGraw B, Smith ML. Meta-analysis in Social Research. Beverly Hills, Calif.: Sage Publications, 1981.

25. Goldsmith JR, Beeser S. Strategies for pooling data in occupational epidemiological studies. Annals: Academy of Medicine (Singapore) 1984;13(suppl 2):297–307.

26. Sacks HS, Chalmers TC, Berk AA et al. Should mild hypertension be treated? An attempted meta-analysis of the clinical trials. Mount Sinai Journal of Medicine 1985;52:265–270.

27. Hunter JE, Schmidt FL, Jackson GB. Meta-analysis: Cumulating Research Findings Across Studies. Beverly Hills, Calif.: Sage Publications, 1982.

28. Klitgaard RF. Identifying exceptional performers. Policy Analysis 1978;4:529–547.

29. Hedges LV, Olkin I. Statistical Methods for Meta-analysis. Orlando, Fla.: Academic Press, 1985.

30. Pillemer DB, Light RJ. Synthesizing extremes: How to use research evidence from many studies. Harvard Educational Review 1980;50:176–195.

31. Proceedings of the Workshop on Methodologic Issues in Overviews of Randomized Clinical Trials. Statistics in Medicine 1987;6:217–409.

32. L'Abbe KA, Detsky AS, O'Rourke K. Meta-analysis in clinical research. Annals of Internal Medicine 1987;107:224–233.

33. Himel HN, Liberati A, Gelber RD et al. Adjuvant chemotherapy for breast cancer: A pooled estimate based on published randomized control trials. Journal of the

American Medical Association 1986;256:1148–1159.

34. Mumford E, Schlesinger HJ, Glass GV. The effects of psychological intervention on recovery from surgery and heart attacks: An analysis of the literature. American Journal of Public Health 1982;72:141–151.

35. Ottenbacher K, Difabio RP. Efficacy of spinal manipulation/mobilization therapy: A meta-analysis. Spine 1985;10:833–837.

36. Tran ZV, Weltman A. Differential effects of exercise on serum lipid and lipoprotein levels seen with changes in body weight: A meta-analysis. Journal of the American Medical Association 1985;254:919–924.

37. Christensen E, Juhl E, Tygstrup N. Treatment of duodenal ulcer: Randomized clinical trials of a decade (1964 to 1974). Gastroenterology 1977;73:1170–1178.

38. Louis TA, Fineberg HV, Mosteller F. Findings for public health from meta-analysis. Annual Review of Public Health 1985;6:1–20.

39. Gilbert JP, McPeek B, Mosteller F. Progress in surgery and anesthesia: Benefits and risks of innovative therapy. In Bunker JP, Barnes BA, Mosteller F (eds). Costs, Risks, and Benefits of Surgery. New York: Oxford University Press, 1977: 124–169.

40. Chalmers TC, Matta RJ, Smith H Jr et al. Evidence favoring the use of anticoagulants in the hospital phase of acute myocardial infarction. New England Journal of Medicine 19;297:1091–1096.

41. Stewart AL, Reynolds EOR, Lipscomb AP. Outcome for infants of very low birthweight: Survey of world literature. Lancet 1981;1:1038–1041.

42. Baum ML, Anish DS, Chalmers TC et al. A survey of clinical trials of antibiotic prophlaxis in colon surgery: Evidence against further use of no-treatment controls. New England Journal of Medicine 1981;305:795–799.

43. Blackburn BA, Smith H, Chalmers TC. The inadequate evidence for short hospital stay after hernia for varicose vein stripping surgery. Mount Sinai Journal of Medicine 1982;49:383–390.

44. Stamfer MJ, Goldhaber SZ, Yusuf S et al. Effect of intravenous streptokinase on acute myocardial infarction. New England Journal of Medicine 1982;307:1180–1182.

45. Toth PJ, Horwitz RI. Conflicting clinical trials and the uncertainty of treating mild hypertension. American Journal of Medicine 1983;75:482–488.

46. Thacker SB. Quality of controlled clinical trials: The case of imaging ultrasound in obstetrics: A review. British Journal of Obstetrics and Gynaecology 1985;92:437–444.

47. Colditz GA, Tuden RL, Oster G. Rates of venous thrombosis after general surgery: Combined results of randomized clinical trials. Lancet 1986;2:143–146.

48. Eddy DM. The use of confidence profiles to assess tissue-type plasminogen activator. In Califf RM, Wagner GS (eds). Acute Coronary Care 1987. Boston: Martinus Nijhoff, 1986, chap 7.

49. Schneider AP II. Breast milk jaundice in the newborn: A real entity. Journal of the American Medical Association 1986;255:3270–3274.

50. Banta HD, Thacker SB. Assessing the costs and benefits of electronic fetal monitoring. Obstetrical and Gynecological Survey 1979;34:627–642.

51. Thacker SB. The efficacy of intrapartum electronic fetal monitoring. American Journal of Obstetrics and Gynecology 1987;156:24–30.

52. MacDonald D, Grant A, Sheridan-Pereira M et al. The Dublin randomized con-

trolled trial of intrapartum fetal heart rate monitoring. American Journal of Obstetrics and Gynecology 1985;152:524–539.

53. Chalmers I. Randomized controlled trials of intrapartum monitoring, in Thalhammer O, Baumgarten KV, Pollack A (eds). Perinatal Medicine. Stuttgart, West Germany: Georg Thieme Verlag, 1979:260–265.

54. Leveno KJ, Cunningham FG, Nelson S, et al. A prospective comparison of selective and universal electronic fetal monitoring in 34,995 pregnancies. New England Journal of Medicine 1986;315:615–619.

55. Luthy DA, Shy KK, Van Bell G et al. A randomized trial of electronic fetal monitoring in premature labor. Obstetrics and Gynecology 1987;69:687–695.

56. Eysenck HJ. An exercise in mega-silliness. American Psychologist 1978;33:517.

57. Eysenck HJ. Meta-analysis: An abuse of research integration. Journal of Special Education 1984;18:41–59.

58. Taveggia TC. Resolving research controversy through empirical cumulation. Sociological Methods and Research 1974;2:395–407.

59. Chalmers TC, Levin H, Sacks HS et al. Meta-analysis of clinical trials as a scientific discipline: I. Control of bias and comparison with large cooperative trials. Statistics in Medicine 1987;6:315–325.

60. Chalmers TC, Berrier J, Sacks HS et al. Meta-analysis of clinical trials as a scientific discipline: II. Replicate variability and comparison of studies that agree and disagree. Statistics in Medicine 1987;6:733–744.

61. DerSimonian R, Laird N. Meta-analysis in clinical trials. Controlled Clinical Trials 1986;7:177–188.

62. Mintz J. Integrating research evidence: A commentary on meta-analysis. 1983;51:71–75.

63. Cook TD, Leviton LC. Reviewing the literature: A comparison of traditional methods with meta-analysis. Journal of Personality 1980;48:449–472.

64. Cooper HM, Arkin RM. On quantitative reviewing. Journal of Personality 1981;49:225–230.

65. Wilson GT, Rachman SJ. Meta-analysis and the evaluation of psychotherapy outcome: Limitations and liabilities. Journal of Consulting and Clinical Psychology 1983;51:54–64.

66. Sacks HS, Berrier J, Reitman D et al. Meta-analysis of randomized controlled trials. New England Journal of Medicine 1987;316:450–455.

67. Light RJ, Pillemer DB. Numbers and narrative: Combining their strengths in research reviews. Harvard Educational Review 1982;52:1–26.

68. Cooper HM, Rosenthal R. Statistical versus traditional procedures for summarizing research findings. Psychological Bulletin 1980;87:442–449.

69. Bissonnette JM. Relationship between continuous fetal heart rate patterns and Apgar score in the newborn. British Journal of Obstetrics and Gynaecology 1975;82:24–28.

70 Gabert HA, Stenchever MA. Continuous electronic monitoring of fetal heart rate during labor. American Journal of Obstetrics and Gynecology 1973;115:919–923.

71. Schifrin BS, Dame L. Fetal heart rate patterns, prediction of Apgar score. Journal of the American Medical Association 1972;219:1322–1325.

72. Saldana LR, Schulman H, Yang W. Electronic fetal monitoring during labor. Obstetrics and Gynecology 1976;47:706–710.

73. Tipton R, Shelley T. An index of fetal welfare in labour. Journal of Obstetrics and Gynaecology of the British Commonwealth 1971;78:702–706.

9

An Introduction to a Bayesian Method for Meta-Analysis: The Confidence Profile Method[*]

DAVID M. EDDY, VIC HASSELBLAD, and ROSS SHACHTER

The Confidence Profile Method is a form of meta-analysis. It is a Bayesian method for interpreting, adjusting, and combining evidence to estimate a probability distribution for a parameter. Examples of parameters are health outcomes, economic outcomes, and variables that might be used in models, such as the sensitivity of a diagnostic test or the prevalence of a risk factor.

This paper introduces some of the mathematics, indicates the scope of the method, and gives a few examples of formulas. Additional information can be found in Eddy (1); Eddy, Hasselblad, and Shachter (2); and Shachter, Eddy, and Hasselblad (3).

BASIC FORMULAS

Let ε be the parameter of interest. Designate as X_1 the results of a piece of evidence about ε, say, the results of an experiment. Our task is to estimate the distribution for ε, conditional on the results of the experiment, X_1. Using the conventional notation for a conditional probability, we denote this distribution as $\pi(\varepsilon \mid X_1)$. By Bayes's formula, this posterior distribution is calculated as the product of a prior distribution for ε [which we denote as $\pi(\varepsilon)$] and the likelihood function for the experiment.

$$\pi(\varepsilon \mid X_1) = k \, L(X_1 \mid \varepsilon) \, \pi(\varepsilon) \tag{1}$$

[*]This paper was previously published in Medical Decision Making 1990;10:15-23.

The likelihood function, $L(X_1 | \varepsilon)$, gives the likelihood of observing the actual results of the experiment (X_1), conditional on any possible value of the true effect of the technology (ε). "k" is a normalizing constant.

Equation 1 is quite general. A specific example is the formula for analyzing the effect of a single diagnostic test on the probability that a patient has a disease.

$$P(\text{Disease} | \text{Test Pos}) = \frac{1}{P(\text{Test Pos})} P(\text{Test Pos} | \text{Disease}) P(\text{Disease})$$

The "predictive value positive" [P(Disease | Test Positive)] corresponds to the posterior distribution, the sensitivity of the test [P(Test Positive | Disease)] corresponds to the likelihood function, the prior probability of disease [P(Disease)] corresponds to the prior distribution, and the denominator [P(Test Positive)] corresponds to the normalizing constant.

Now suppose a second piece of evidence gives results X_2. The updated posterior distribution for ε that incorporates both pieces of evidence can be calculated by inserting its likelihood function in the equation.

$$\pi(\varepsilon | X_1, X_2) = k \, L_2(X_2 | \varepsilon, X_1) L_1(X_1 | \varepsilon) \, \pi(\varepsilon) \tag{2}$$

If the experiments are dependent, the likelihood function for the second experiment is conditional on the results of the first experiment, as shown in Equation 2. If the experiments are independent, which is very frequently the case, then:

$$L_2(X_2 | \varepsilon, X_1) = L_2(X_2 | \varepsilon)$$

and:

$$\pi(\varepsilon | X_1, X_2) = k \, L_2(X_2 | \varepsilon) L_1(X_1 | \varepsilon) \, \pi(\varepsilon) \tag{3}$$

Biases

An important problem in the evaluation of evidence is the presence of biases. An important difference between the Confidence Profile Method and other meta-analysis techniques is the explicit modeling of biases and their incorporation in the distribution for the parameter of interest. Again designate ε as the parameter of interest. For a variety of reasons, a particular experiment might estimate a related but slightly different parameter. Call this ε' or the "study parameter." If the study parameter is not identical to the parameter of interest (i.e., if $\varepsilon \neq \varepsilon'$), the evidence is biased.

A wide variety of factors can bias an experiment. For example, biases to internal validity of a two-arm prospective controlled trial include:

- Inaccurate measurement of outcomes
- Incorrect determination of who actually received a technology
- Crossover: some patients who are offered a technology might not receive

it ("dilution") and some patients in the control group might receive it anyway ("contamination")

- Differences in the patients in the two groups ("patient-selection bias")
- Loss of patients to follow-up, and
- Uncertainty about the actual number of cases or outcomes.

Biases to external validity include:

- Differences between the population involved in the experiment and the population of interest
- Differences between the technology used in the experiment and the technology of interest (e.g., type of equipment, dose of a drug, skill of practitioners)
- Differences in follow-up times across experiments, and
- Differences in effect measures across experiments.

If biases exist, indiscriminate use of meta-analytic methods that fail to adjust for them will be incorrect. In the case of the Bayesian approach, if an experiment contains biases to internal validity, the likelihood function will apply to ε' rather than ε. That is,

$$\pi(\varepsilon \mid X) \neq L (X \mid \varepsilon') \, \pi(\varepsilon)$$

The Confidence Profile Method can correct for this by defining a function that relates the study parameter (ε') to the parameter of interest (ε). Call this function: $f(\varepsilon)$. This function can be substituted for ε' in the likelihood function, restoring the correctness of Bayes's formula.

$$\pi(\varepsilon \mid X) = L[X \mid f(\varepsilon)] \, \pi(\varepsilon)$$

This last formula illustrates the three basic ingredients of the Confidence Profile Method. The method requires prior distributions, likelihood functions, and functions that describe biases. It also requires functions that define the measures of effect (which will be introduced below).

Prior Distributions

The most conservative and widely used approach uses noninformative prior distributions. The choice of a prior distribution then has a minimal effect on the posterior distribution. Berger (4) has described methods for determining noninformative prior distributions, depending on the interval over which the parameter of interest is defined. For parameters defined on the entire real line $\theta \in (-\infty, \infty)$ the appropriate prior distribution is $\pi(\theta) = 1$. For parameters defined on the positive real line, $\theta \in (0, \infty)$, the appropriate prior is $\pi(\theta) = 1/\theta$. For probabilities defined on the interval $(0,1)$, the method of Jeffreys (5) gives beta distribution with parameters $1/2$, $1/2$. For the multinomial model, the comparable prior for the $\theta_i \in (0,1)$ is a Dirichlet distribution with parameters $1/2, 1/2, \ldots 1/2$.

Likelihood Functions

At the heart of the Confidence Profile Method are likelihood functions. A different likelihood function is needed for each type of experiment, each type of outcome, and each type of effect measure. The possible combinations are shown in Table 9.1.

TABLE 9.1 Likelihood functions for various types of experimental designs, outcomes, and effect measures

	Outcomes			
Designs	Dichotomous	Categorical	Count	Continuous
One-Arm Prospective	Rate	Rate Score	Mean Count	Mean Score Median Score
Two-Arm Prospective	Difference Ratio Odds Ratio % Difference	Difference Ratio	Difference Ratio	Difference Ratio
n-Arm Prospective	Coefficients of Logistic Regression Equation, β_i	Coefficients of Linear Regression Equation, β_i	Coefficients of Linear Regression Equation, β_i	Coefficients of Linear Regression Equation, β_i
2×2 Case Control	Odds Ratio	NA	NA	NA
$2 \times n$ Case Control	Coefficients of Logistic Regression Equation, β_i	NA	NA	NA
Matched Case Control	Odds Ratio	NA	NA	NA
Cross Sectional	Coefficients of Logistic Regression Equation, β_i	Coefficients of Linear Regression Equation, β_i	Coefficients of Linear Regression Equation, β_i	Coefficients of Linear Regression Equation, β_i

NA, not applicable.

TABLE 9.2 Results of a hypothetical randomized controlled clinical trial

| Study | | Controls | | Treated | |
No.	Design	No.	Survive	No.	Survive
1	RCT	100	53	104	72

There are four basic outcomes: dichotomous, categorical, counts, and continuous. There is also a large number of experimental designs, including one-arm prospective trials (e.g., clinical series), two-arm prospective trials (e.g., randomized and non-randomized controlled trials), multi-arm prospective trials (e.g., multi-dose drug trials), 2×2 case control studies, $2 \times n$ case control studies, matched case control studies, and cross-sectional studies. Finally, there are a variety of measures of effect. For example, in a two-arm controlled trial involving dichotomous outcomes, the effect of the intervention can be measured as the difference in rates of the outcomes in the two groups, the ratio of rates, the odds ratio, and the percent difference. For case control studies, the measure of effect usually is the odds ratio. For multi-arm prospective studies, $2 \times n$ case control studies, and cross-sectional studies, the parameters of interest might be the coefficients of a logistic regression equation, and so forth. The Confidence Profile Method includes likelihood functions for each type of outcome, experimental design, and effect measure (2).

ILLUSTRATION

Imagine a randomized controlled trial with 100 patients in the control group and 104 patients in the group offered treatment (see Table 9.2). Imagine that 53 of the patients in the control group survive five years, compared with 72 patients in the treatment group. Suppose we are interested in the probability that the difference in survival resulted from the treatment. That is, let ε be the difference in survival rates in the two groups.

To derive the appropriate likelihood function for the difference in survival, we begin by looking at the outcomes in each group. Let θ_c be the true survival rate in the control group, let θ_t be the true survival rate in the treated group, and let ε be the difference in rates caused by treatment, $\varepsilon = \theta_t - \theta_c$.

A joint likelihood function for θ_c and θ_t based on observing 53 survivors of 100 patients in the control group and 72 survivors of 104 patients in the treated group can be derived from the binomial distribution.

$$L(53 \text{ of } 100, 72 \text{ of } 104 \mid \theta_c, \theta_t) \propto \theta_c^{53} (1 - \theta_c)^{47} \theta_t^{72} (1 - \theta_t)^{32}$$

The probability of success in the control group (θ_c) is raised to the power of the observed number of successes in the control group (53), and so forth. Using the definition of $\varepsilon = \theta_t - \theta_c$, we can solve for θ_t in terms of ε and θ_c, and substitute to obtain a joint likelihood for θ_c and ε.

$$L(53 \text{ of } 100, 72 \text{ of } 104 \mid \theta_c, \varepsilon) \propto \theta_c^{53} (1 - \theta_c)^{47} (\varepsilon + \theta_c)^{72} (1 - \varepsilon - \theta_c)^{32}$$

The likelihood function for ε can be obtained by integrating over θ_c (6,7), using a beta distribution with parameters $\alpha = 1/2$, $\beta = 1/2$ as a noninformative prior for θ_c.

$$L(53 \text{ of } 100, 72 \text{ of } 104 \mid \varepsilon)$$
$$\propto \int \theta_c^{53} (1 - \theta_c)^{47} (\varepsilon + \theta_c)^{72} (1 - \varepsilon - \theta_c)^{32} \, \beta_{1/2, 1/2}(\theta_c) \, d(\theta_c) \qquad (4)$$

This likelihood function can be used in Bayes's formula to calculate a posterior distribution for ε. The result is illustrated in Figure 9.1.

The horizontal axis shows the range of possible values for ε. Because θ_c and θ_t can each range from 0 to 1, the range of ε, which is $\theta_t - \theta_c$, is from -1 to $+1$. In this case the distribution for ε is centered approximately over 0.16, indicating that treatment increases the probability of survival by approximately 16 percent. The uncertainty about that estimate is indicated by the shape of the distribution.

From this distribution it is easy to calculate the probability that the true effect, ε, lies between any set of limits the assessor cares to specify. The distribution itself can be used directly in any additional calculations the assessor cares to perform (e.g., decision trees, mathematical models).

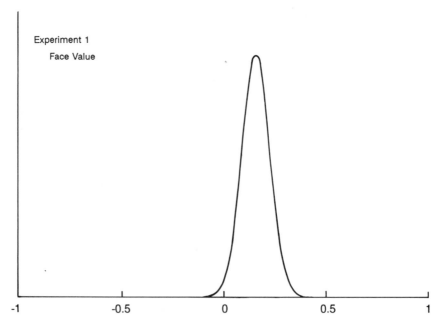

FIGURE 9.1 Probability distribution A for an increase in five-year survival as a result of treatment. Based on a randomized controlled trial of 204 patients.

TABLE 9.3 Results of a hypothetical randomized controlled clinical trial with dilution

Study No.	Design	Controls No.	Controls Survive	Treated No.	Treated Survive	Biases
1	RCT	100	53	104	72	Dilution 20%

Now, suppose there is a bias in this trial. Suppose the best available information indicates that 20 percent of the patients offered the treatment did not get it. That is, there is a dilution bias of approximately 20 percent (see Table 9.3).

If that is true, the likelihood function just derived (Equation 4) no longer estimates the parameter of interest, i.e., the effect of treatment in people who actually *receive* treatment. Rather, the trial estimates a different parameter, ε', which is the effectiveness of *offering treatment in the setting of the trial*.

$$L(53 \text{ of } 100, 72 \text{ of } 104 \mid \varepsilon') = \int \theta_c^{53} (1 - \theta_c)^{47}(\varepsilon' + \theta_c)^{72}(1 - \varepsilon' - \theta_c)^{32}$$
$$\beta^{1/2,1/2}(\theta_c) \, d(\theta_c) \tag{5}$$

This likelihood function cannot be used for ε in Equation 1 without further work.

To adjust for this dilution, we need a model for how dilution affects the results of the trial. As before, let θ_t be the true probability of survival in people who actually receive treatment. Let θ_t' be the true probability of survival in the people who are offered treatment in the trial. Finally, let α be the fraction of people who are offered treatment but do not receive it. In that case, the probability of survival in patients *offered* treatment, θ_t', is the probability of survival in people who actually *receive* treatment, θ_t, multiplied by the proportion who do receive treatment, $(1 - \alpha)$, plus the probability of survival in people who do not receive treatment, θ_c, multiplied by the proportion who do not receive it, α.

$$\theta_t' = (1 - \alpha)\theta_t + \alpha\theta_c$$

If the dilution is thought to be 20 percent, set α to 0.2 to obtain a formula for θ_t' in terms of θ_t and θ_c

$$\theta_t' = 0.8\theta_t + 0.2\theta_c$$

Substituting for θ_t' in the formula for the effect measured by the experiment, $\varepsilon' = \theta_t' - \theta_c$ implies that the dilution causes ε' to be equal to 0.8ε.

The formula for ε' can then be substituted in the right side of Equation 5 to obtain a likelihood function in terms of ε, the parameter of interest.

$$L(53 \text{ of } 100, 72 \text{ of } 104 \mid \varepsilon) = \int \theta_c^{53} (1 - \theta_c)^{47}(0.8\varepsilon + \theta_c)^{72}(1 - 0.8\varepsilon - \theta_c)^{32}$$
$$\beta^{1/2,1/2}(\theta_c) \, d(\theta_c) \tag{6}$$

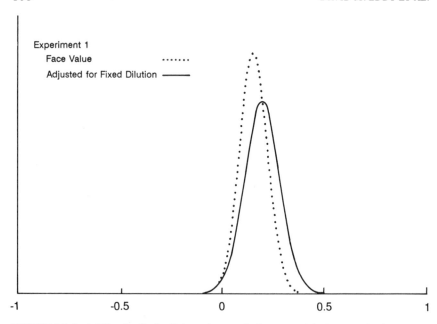

FIGURE 9.2 Probability distribution B for an increase in five-year survival as a result of treatment. Based on a randomized controlled trial of 204 patients in which 20 percent of the patients offered treatment did not actually receive treatment (dilution bias of 20 percent).

Use of this "adjusted" likelihood function in Bayes's formula results in a posterior distribution that corrects for the bias (see Figure 9.2). The result is shown as the solid line in the figure, which includes for comparison the original distribution that took the experiment at face value, without adjusting for dilution. The presence of dilution caused the experiment to underestimate the true effect of the treatment in patients who actually receive treatment; the best estimate is now a 20 percent increase in survival for people who receive treatment.

Now suppose we are uncertain about the magnitude of dilution. Suppose all we can say is that we are 95 percent confident that the proportion of patients offered treatment who did not receive it (α) is between 6 percent and 42 percent (see Table 9.4).

TABLE 9.4 Results of a hypothetical randomized controlled clinical trial with dilution and uncertainty

Study No.	Design	Controls No.	Controls Survive	Treated No.	Treated Survive	Biases
1	RCT	100	53	104	72	Dilution 20% (6 – 42%)

This uncertainty can be incorporated in the likelihood function by using a distribution for α [say, $\beta_{a,b}(\alpha)$] and integrating over that distribution.

$$L(53 \text{ of } 100, 72 \text{ of } 104 \mid \varepsilon) =$$
$$\iint \theta_c^{53}(1-\theta_c)^{47}(0.8\varepsilon+\theta_c)^{72}(1-0.8\varepsilon-\theta_c)^{32}\,\beta_{1/2,1/2}(\theta_c)\,\beta_{a,b}(\alpha)\,d\theta\,d_c\alpha$$

The result is shown in Figure 9.3. The dotted line represents the posterior distribution if the study is taken at face value; the dashed line takes into account a dilution factor of 0.2; the solid line incorporates uncertainty about the magnitude of that dilution.

Additional biases and nested biases can be incorporated in the analysis. For example, in addition to dilution, there might be errors in measurement of outcomes (e.g., there might be a 5 percent probability that a patient in the control group labeled as dead from the disease actually died of other causes). Or we might suspect that patients who dilute from the group offered treatment have an inherently lower risk of the outcome. Or some who dilute might have gotten a modified treatment that was, say, halfway between the treatment offered the "treated" and control groups. As in the illustration, it is possible to incorporate uncertainty about any parameter used to define a bias.

Now consider a second experiment that has 50 patients in the control group with 23 survivors, and 50 patients in the group offered treatment with 38 survivors (see Table 9.5).

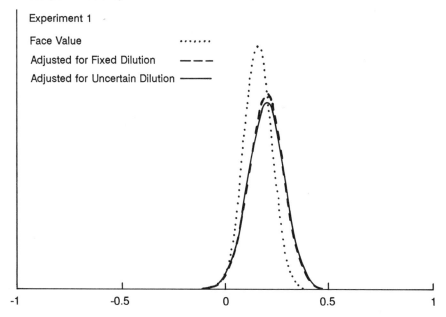

FIGURE 9.3 Probability distribution C for an increase in five-year survival as a result of treatment. Based on a randomized controlled trial of 204 patients assuming (1) no biases (dotted line), (2) dilution bias of 20 percent (dashed line), and (3) dilution bias of uncertain magnitude (solid line).

TABLE 9.5 Results of two hypothetical randomized controlled clinical trials

Study No.	Design	Controls No.	Survive	Treated No.	Survive	Biases
1	RCT	100	53	104	72	Dilution 20% (6 – 42%)
2	RCT	50	23	50	38	None

Suppose there are no biases in this experiment. The likelihood function for this experiment $[L_2(X_2 \mid \epsilon)]$ is also based on the binomial distribution and is derived in the same fashion as for the first experiment (Equation 4). The results are indicated in Figure 9.4, which includes for comparison the first study, after adjustment for dilution (the dotted line).

Bayes's formula can be used to combine the information in the two experiments to derive a new posterior distribution (Equation 3). This distribution is shown as the solid line in Figure 9.5, with the distributions for the two individual studies shown as the dashed lines.

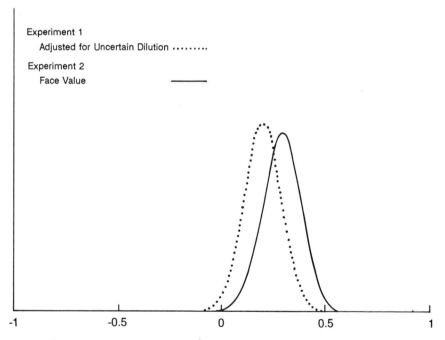

FIGURE 9.4 Probability distribution D for an increase in five-year survival as a result of treatment. Based on a randomized controlled trial of 1,000 patients (solid line), compared with a randomized controlled trial of 204 patients adjusted for dilution bias (dotted line).

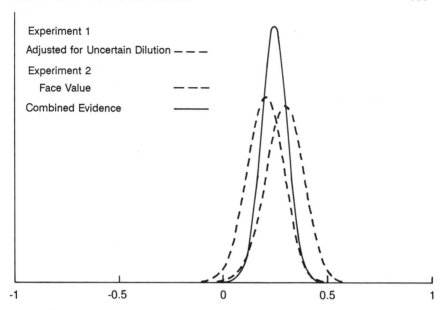

Experiment 1
Adjusted for Uncertain Dilution — — —
Experiment 2
Face Value   — — —
Combined Evidence   ———

-1   -0.5   0   0.5   1

FIGURE 9.5 Probability distribution E for an increase in five-year survival as a result of treatment. Based on the combined results of two randomized controlled trials (solid line). The probability distributions based on the results of the individual randomized controlled trials are shown as dashed lines.

BASIC FORMULAS IN THE CONFIDENCE PROFILE METHOD

The Confidence Profile Method contains likelihood functions for all the experimental designs, outcome measures, and effect measures shown in Table 9.1 (2). There is no requirement that all the studies to be combined have the same design. In general, likelihood functions for studies with dichotomous outcomes are based on the binomial distribution; those with categorical outcomes are based on the multinomial distribution; those with counts are based on the Poisson distribution; and those with continuous outcomes are based on the normal distribution. This paper illustrated one likelihood function: a two-arm prospective study with dichotomous outcomes, whose effect is measured as the difference in rates of outcomes. The Confidence Profile Method also contains models for all the biases listed previously (1, 2), one of which (dilution) was illustrated in this paper. It also incorporates models for compound or nested biases (2).

ADDITIONAL FORMULAS

The Confidence Profile Method contains a number of formulas for handling problems that are more complex than the ones just described. These include a hierarchical Bayes method, formulas for analyzing indirect evidence, and formulas for analyzing technology families.

Hierarchical Bayes

The hierarchical Bayes method addresses the following problem. Again, let ϵ be the true effect in which we are interested. However, it is possible that Mother Nature does not have a single particular value for this effect. For example, the success rate of a surgical procedure might be slightly different in New York than in Chicago, due to factors that we cannot identify or adjust for explicitly. In such cases, it is reasonable to act as though Mother Nature has a *distribution* for the true effect; our task is to estimate the distribution. The hierarchical Bayes method accomplishes that (8). An analogous approach using classical statistical techniques (called the "random effects model") has been described by DerSimonian and Laird (9).

Indirect Evidence

The problem posed by indirect evidence is that experiments frequently relate a technology (e.g., exercise), not to the health outcomes in which we are really interested (e.g., a heart attack), but to an intermediate outcome (e.g., blood pressure, obesity, or serum cholesterol). Another body of evidence must then be used to relate the intermediate outcomes to health outcomes.

Diagram of indirect evidence:

Technology $\rightarrow$ Intermediate Outcomes $\rightarrow$ Health Outcomes

The Confidence Profile Method includes formulas for combining the two bodies of evidence, including the possibility that the intermediate outcome is not a perfect indicator of the health outcome (1). For example, exercise might have an independent effect on the chance of a heart attack not mediated through a change in serum cholesterol.

Technology Families

The formulas for analyzing technology families address another common problem of technology assessment. Frequently, there are a variety of technologies for the same health problem. For example, breast cancer can be treated with many different combinations of surgery, radiation, chemotherapy, and hormonal therapy. A review of the literature might uncover studies that relate many pairs of technologies, represented as the solid lines in Figure 9.6, but not all. For example, suppose we are interested in comparing technology B with technology E, as indicated by the dashed line in Figure 9.6. Even though there is no direct evidence for this comparison, it is possible to compare these two technologies using information about other technologies that *have* been compared. The Confidence Profile Method contains formulas for accomplishing that (1).

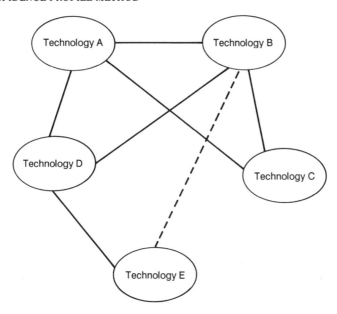

FIGURE 9.6 Diagram of technology families. Solid lines indicate the existence of trials relating two technologies; dashed line indicates the two technologies to be compared.

Research Planning

The posterior distribution for the parameter of interest, estimated from existing information, can be used as a prior distribution for calculating the probability that future experiments of various types (e.g., different designs, different sample sizes) will yield certain results. The simplest example arises when calculating the power of an experiment. Power calculations require postulation of a particular magnitude of effect; the formulas calculate the probability of a statistically significant result at a specified level of significance, conditional on the assumed magnitude of the effect. The distribution for the effect calculated by the Confidence Profile Method can be used in these calculations to obtain a power conditional on the existing evidence for the effect, rather than a hypothesized effect. Because the Confidence Profile Method delivers a distribution, it can also calculate the probability an experiment will yield results within a specified range (rather than simply a statistically significant result, as in a power calculation). For example, the Confidence Profile Method can be used to estimate the probability that a third randomized controlled trial with 100 patients in each group will show that treatment increases survival between 15 percent and 25 percent, taking into account the evidence from the first two trials.

Additional techniques in the Confidence Profile Method enable calculation of the covariance matrix for all parameters incorporated in the analysis. For example, the covariance matrix indicates how a change in the variance of the distribution for α, the dilution in the first experiment, affects the posterior distribution for the parameter of interest. This feature enables calculation of the sensitivity of the result to the magnitude and range of uncertainty about any parameters used in the calculations.

IMPLEMENTATION

To apply the method a problem must be formulated in a way that uses these ingredients accurately and efficiently, and a solution must be calculated. There are two basic approaches, which we call the stepwise approach and the integrated approach. The stepwise approach, described in this paper, basically consists of evaluating one experiment at a time, adjusting each to ensure that it estimates the parameter of interest, and combining them according to Bayes's formula. This approach works well for problems that are relatively straightforward. For more complex assessment problems, the Confidence Profile Method uses an integrated approach that takes into account the multivariate nature of many assessment problems, with dependencies between parameters, biases, and pieces of evidence. The integrated approach is extremely powerful, although more difficult to conceptualize (5). Both approaches involve considerable mathematics.

We are producing a number of aids to help make the Confidence Profile Method available. These include a book that pulls all the information together, with examples; software that implements the stepwise approach; and a computer-based, interactive tutorial that will lead a novice through a complete exposition of the method.

RELATIONSHIP TO OTHER META-ANALYSIS TECHNIQUES

The Confidence Profile Method differs from meta-analysis techniques based on classical statistics in several important ways. First, because it is based on Bayesian statistics, the Confidence Profile Method gives marginal probability distributions for the parameters of interest and, if the integrated approach is used, a joint probability distribution for all the parameters. Other meta-analysis techniques calculate a point estimate for a single effect measure and confidence intervals for the estimate under an assumption of large sample sizes. The value of probability distributions is that they can be used to calculate the probability that the "true value" of a parameter lies within any specified range. Probability distributions also can be used in models of varying complexity, including simple transformations (e.g., logs, powers), simple operations (e.g., addition, subtraction by convolution), decision trees, and stochastic models (e.g., Markov chains).

A second distinguishing feature is that the Confidence Profile Method allows the assessor to derive probability distributions for parameters that are functions of other parameters. Classical meta-analysis, as currently formulated, enables one to combine evidence about a single parameter. For example, the production of probability distributions enables the Confidence Profile Method to analyze indirect evidence and technology families, neither of which can be analyzed by other meta-analysis techniques.

A third distinguishing feature of the Confidence Profile Method, again enabled by the use of Bayesian statistics, is the explicit modeling of biases to internal and external validity. Other meta-analysis techniques take biases into account either by a "take it or leave it" approach, or by assigning weights. In the latter approach, the assessor assigns each study a weight designed to decrease its influence compared with the other studies being synthesized. The main problem with this approach is that weights do not accurately correct for the effects of biases. Biases cause a piece of evidence to misestimate the magnitude and range of uncertainty of a parameter. The use of weights assumes the study is correctly estimating the magnitude of the parameter; the effect of the weight is only to modify the variance of the estimate. A second problem with weights is largely due to the first; there is no theoretical basis for estimating the appropriate weights to adjust for a specific bias or collection of biases. In the "take it or leave it" approach, the assessor decides whether to accept a study for inclusion in a synthesis, which is tantamount to assuming it has no biases, or decides to reject it, which is tantamount to assuming its biases invalidate its results. This is equivalent to assigning a weight of either 1 or 0.

In contrast, the Confidence Profile Method models biases explicitly and incorporates the models in the formulas that synthesize the evidence. These models allow the assessor to think about each bias individually, in natural units. For example, an assessor who wants to adjust a randomized controlled trial for dilution describes the proportion of people who "dilute"—who are offered treatment but do not receive it. To estimate the effect of possible errors in measurement of outcomes (e.g., errors in claims data, chart notes, or patient recall), the assessor can describe the applicable error rates. The estimates of the magnitudes of biases can be based on records, separate experiments, or if necessary, subjective judgments. The Confidence Profile Method also allows for the nesting of biases and dependencies between biases. Finally, the method enables the assessor to describe uncertainty about the magnitude of any bias. Uncertainty can be present if a bias is estimated empirically, due to the inherent imprecision of the experiment (e.g., sample size), or if a bias must be estimated subjectively.

The ability of the Confidence Profile Method to incorporate subjective judgments about biases is one example of its third important feature, which is to provide a formal, axiomatically based method for incorporating subjective judgments in a meta-analysis.

The fourth main difference that distinguishes the Confidence Profile Method from other meta-analysis methods is that it is a unified set of techniques. The assessor can describe a system of equations that incorporates simultaneously all the basic parameters (e.g., population parameters), functional parameters (parameters that are functions of other parameters), experimental evidence, and subjective judgments. This enables the assessor to represent the multivariate nature of the assessment problem, taking into account dependencies between variables and pieces of evidence, and functional relationships as complicated as the assessor cares to define. The solution of the system of equations yields a joint probability distribution for all the parameters.

SUMMARY

To summarize, the Confidence Profile Method can be used to assess technologies when the available evidence involves a variety of experimental designs, types of outcomes, and effect measures; a variety of biases; combinations of biases and nested biases; uncertainty about biases; an underlying variability in the parameter of interest; indirect evidence; and technology families. The result of an analysis with the Confidence Profile Method is a posterior distribution for the parameter of interest, posterior distributions for other parameters, and a covariance matrix for all the parameters in the model. The posterior distributions incorporate all the uncertainty the assessor chooses to describe about any parameter used in the analysis.

REFERENCES

1. Eddy DM. The Confidence Profile Method: A Bayesian method for assessing health technologies. Operations Research 1989;37:210–228.
2. Eddy DM, Hasselblad V, Shachter R. A Bayesian method for synthesizing evidence: The Confidence Profile Method. International Journal of Technology Assessment in Health Care, in press.
3. Shachter R, Eddy DM, Hasselblad V. An influence diagram approach to the Confidence Profile Method for health technology assessment. Technical Report, Center for Health Policy Research and Education, Duke University, Durham, N.C., 1988.
4. Berger JO. Statistical Decision Theory and Bayesian Analysis. New York: Springer-Verlag, 1985.
5. Jeffreys H. Theory of Probability. London: Oxford University Press, 1961.
6. Basu D. On the elimination of nuisance parameters. Journal of the American Statistical Association 1977;72:355–366.
7. Berger J, Wolpert R. The Likelihood Principle (2nd edition). Hayward, Calif.: Institute of Mathematical Statistics, 1988.
8. Wolpert RL, Hasselblad V, Eddy DM. Hierarchical Bayes methods for confidence profiles. Technical Report, Center for Health Policy Research and Education, Duke University, Durham, N.C., 1987.
9. DerSimonian R, Laird NM. Meta-analysis in clinical trials. Controlled Clinical Trials 1986;7:177–188.

10

Should We Change the Rules for Evaluating Medical Technologies?

DAVID M. EDDY

Before we launch a new medical technology, we would like to show that it satisfies four criteria:

- It improves the health outcomes patients care about—pain, death, anxiety, disfigurement, disability.
- Its benefits outweigh its harms.
- Its health effects are worth its costs.
- And, if resources are limited, it deserves priority over other technologies.

To apply any of these criteria we need to estimate the magnitude of the technology's benefits and harms. We want to gather this information as accurately, quickly, and inexpensively as possible to speed the use of technologies that have these properties and direct our energy away from technologies that do not.

There are many ways to estimate a technology's benefits and harms. They range from simply asking experts (pure clinical judgment) to conducting multiple randomized controlled trials, with anecdotes, clinical series, data bases, non-randomized controlled trials, and case-control studies in between. The choice of a method has great influence on the cost of the evaluation, the duration of time required for the evaluation, the accuracy of the information gained, the complexity of administering the evaluation, and the ease of defending the subsequent decisions.

The problem before us is to determine which set of methods delivers information of sufficiently high quality to draw conclusions with confidence, at the lowest cost in time and money.

CURRENT EVALUATIVE METHODS

Currently, very different methods are used to evaluate different types of medical technologies. There are some amazing inconsistencies. In some settings, we insist on direct evidence that compares the effects of the technology against suitable controls, using multiple randomized controlled trials in a variety of settings. In other settings, we do not require *any* direct comparison of the technology and a control, or *any* explicit comparison of the technology's benefits versus its harms or costs.

A good example of the first strategy is the evaluation required by the Food and Drug Administration for approval of drugs. I will never forget my first exposure to a new drug application. It described more than a dozen randomized controlled trials involving about 2,000 patients. It filled a room; consisted of 65,000 pages, which, if stood in a pile, would reach 49.5 $1/2$ feet; cost more than $10 million; required four years to complete; and needed a truck to haul it to Washington. At the other end of the spectrum is the evaluation of medical and surgical procedures. For most, there are no randomized controlled trials at all.

There are even inconsistencies within these categories. For example, we can insist that a pharmaceutical company produce the finest evidence that a drug alters some intermediate outcome (e.g., intraocular pressure), but require no controlled evidence at all that changing the intermediate outcome improves the outcome of real interest to patients (e.g., loss of visual field or blindness). We can require dozens of randomized controlled trials to demonstrate that a drug is effective for a particular indication, and leave it to pure clinical judgment to determine its effectiveness for other indications.

These inconsistencies have tremendous implications for the quality of care, the cost of research, and the time required to get effective innovations into widespread use. Consider just the implications for costs. If we demanded at least two randomized controlled trials for every innovation, research costs would be increased by billions of dollars a year. If we were to accept clinical judgment for every innovation, we could save billions of dollars that we now spend on randomized controlled trials, and speed the introduction of new technologies by years.

Given these inconsistencies and their implications, it is worthwhile to ask what information we are really trying to gather with our system for evaluating medical technologies. That might help us determine the best way to gather it.

WHAT ARE WE TRYING TO LEARN?

We need two things to make decisions about a technology. First, we must estimate the approximate magnitude of its benefits and harms. Second, we must determine the range of uncertainty about the estimates. These two points are so crucial to an understanding of the different methods for evaluating technologies that they are worth discussion.

Suppose the outcome of interest is the probability of dying after a heart attack and the technology is a thrombolytic agent. Suppose an experiment has been conducted with 400 patients randomly allocated to receive either the treatment (200 patients) or a placebo (200 patients). Finally, suppose that during the follow-up period, 20 patients in the placebo group died of heart attacks, while 10 patients in the treated group died. Thus, without treatment, the chance of dying of a heart attack is 20 in 200 or 10 percent; with treatment, the chance of dying of a heart attack is 10 in 200, or 5 percent. The magnitude of the effect of treatment is a 5 percent decrease in the chance of dying of a heart attack (10 percent − 5 percent = 5 percent). This effect is shown as the large arrow in Figure 10.1.

For a variety of reasons (e.g., sample size), there is uncertainty about an estimate of this type. This uncertainty can be displayed in terms of confidence intervals or probability distributions. For this particular example, the 95 percent confidence intervals for the estimated effect of the technology range from 0.2

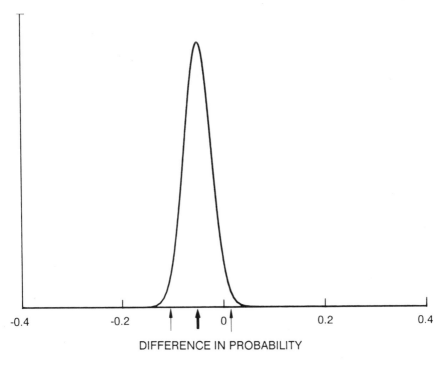

DIFFERENCE IN PROBABILITY

FIGURE 10.1 Results of randomized controlled clinical trial of hypothetical treatment for heart attacks. Best estimates of the effect (large arrow), 95 percent confidence limits (small arrows), and probability distribution of the effect (solid line).

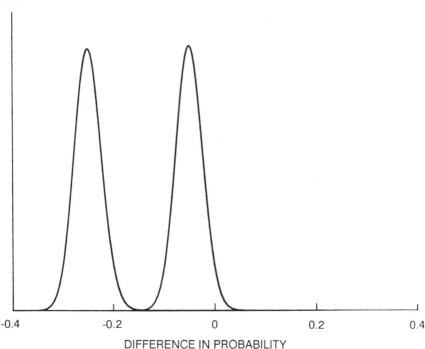

FIGURE 10.2 Probability distributions of effects of two hypothetical treatments for heart attacks. Treatment A (best estimate of effect is –0.05), treatment B (best estimate of effect is – 0.25).

percent to –10.2 percent. These are indicated by the smaller arrows on the graph. The range of uncertainty can also be displayed as a probability distribution for the effect of the technology; it is shown as the solid line. (The height of the distribution at any point reflects the probability that the true reduction in mortality is near that point. Thus, the most likely value for the reduction in mortality is the value under the highest point of the distribution, 5 percent).

Both the estimated magnitude of the technology and the range of uncertainty are important. For example, it makes a big difference whether the technology reduces the chance of dying of a heart attack by 5 percent or by 25 percent (see Figure 10.2). It also makes a big difference whether the range of uncertainty is ±5.2 percent or ±8.3 percent (see Figure 10.3). To people who interpret statistical significance rigidly, there is even a big difference between a range of uncertainty of ±5.2 percent and ±4.9 percent (see Figure 10.4).

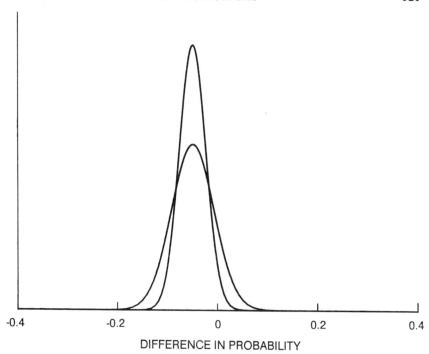

FIGURE 10.3 Probability distributions of effects of a hypothetical treatment for heart attacks as estimated from two randomized controlled clinical trials. Trial A (narrow range of uncertainty), trial B (wider range of uncertainty).

QUALITY OF INFORMATION IN DIFFERENT DESIGNS:
FACE VALUE

All methods for evaluating a technology, from the lowly pure clinical judgment to the lofty randomized controlled trial, provide information on the magnitude of effect and the range of uncertainty. Furthermore, for the empirical methods, if it were reasonable to take each method at face value (i.e., if it were possible to assume that there were no biases to internal or external validity), then *all* the designs, case for case, would be almost equally good at estimating the magnitude and range of uncertainty of an outcome. Stated another way, if all the results could be taken at face value, randomized controlled trials, case for case, would not provide any more precise or certain information than designs that are considered less rigorous, such as non-randomized controlled trials, case-control studies, comparisons of clinical series, or analyses of data bases.

Consider, for example, two studies of breast cancer screening in women over age 50. One was a randomized controlled trial of approximately 100,000 women (58,148 women in the group offered screening and 41,104 women in the

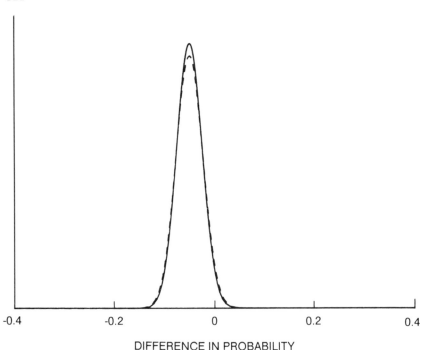

DIFFERENCE IN PROBABILITY

FIGURE 10.4 Probability distributions of effects of a hypothetical treatment for heart attacks as estimated from two randomized controlled clinical trials. Trial A statistically significant (solid line), trial B not statistically significant (dashed line).

control group) (1). After seven years of follow-up, there were 71 breast cancer deaths in the group offered screening and 76 breast cancer deaths in the control group. The other was a case-control study in which 54 cases (women who had died of breast cancer) were matched three to one with 162 controls (women who had not died of breast cancer) (2). Retrospective analysis of screening histories found that 11 of the 54 cases had been screened, compared with 73 of the 162 controls. The probability distributions for the percent reduction in mortality implied by these two studies, taken at face value, are shown in Figure 10.5. The degree of certainty (as indicated by the variance or width of the distribution) is just as high for the case-control study as for the randomized controlled trial. The main determinant of the variance of the estimate is not the total number of people involved in the study (100,000 women in the randomized controlled trial versus 216 in the case-control study), but the number of outcomes of interest that occurred (in this case, breast cancer deaths). The variances in the two studies are similar largely because there were almost as many outcomes in the case-control study (54) as in either group of the randomized controlled trial (71 and 76, respectively).

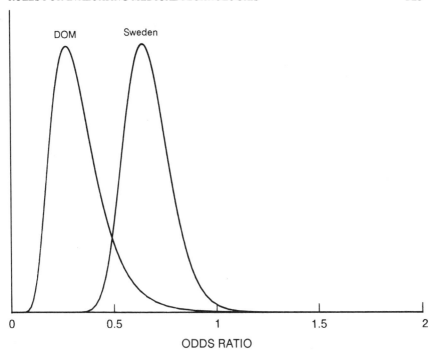

FIGURE 10.5 Probability distributions of two controlled clinical trials of breast cancer screening taken at face value. Swedish prospective RCT; DOM retrospective case-control study (2).

Thus, if we take the two studies at face value, it is clear that they provide virtually the same information. The difference between the studies is logistics. The randomized controlled trial involved recruiting and randomizing 100,000 people, screening about half of them, and following everyone for more than a decade. The logistics of the case-control study, on the other hand, were much simpler and less expensive. It required identifying only 54 women who died of breast cancer (the cases), 162 women matched by year of birth who have not died of breast cancer (the controls), and retrospective ascertainment of which women had been screened. The study collapses down to about 200 women and can be done in six months.

Similar stories can be told about the other designs. Provided the number of cases with the outcome of interest are similar, the degree of certainty in the face value estimates of all the designs will be similar. But the logistics can be vastly different. To push the example to the extreme, if there were a data base that had the pertinent records, the logistics would be as simple as doing the computer runs.

So, if the quality of the information gained by different designs is essentially the same, but the logistics, costs, and time required are very different, the choice of the best design should be quite simple: pick the fastest and least expensive. What is wrong with this picture?

BIASES

The problem, of course, is with the assumption made at the beginning of the story. There we postulated that it was reasonable to take each design at face value—that is, to assume that there were no biases. In fact, there are biases that affect all evaluative methods. Furthermore, the effects of biases determine the rules for evaluating technologies. To solve the problem of choosing the best evaluative methodologies, we need some background on biases.

It is convenient to separate biases into two types. Biases to internal validity affect the accuracy of the results of the study as an estimate of the effect of the technology in the setting in which a study was conducted (e.g., the specific technology, specific patient indications, and so forth). Biases to external validity affect the applicability of the results to other settings (where the techniques, patient indications, and other factors might be different).

Examples of biases to internal validity include patient selection bias, crossover, errors in measurement of outcomes, and errors in ascertainment of exposure to the technology. Patient selection bias exists when patients in the two groups to be compared (e.g., the control and treated groups of a controlled trial) differ in ways that could affect the outcome of interest. When such differences exist, a difference in outcomes could be due at least in part to inherent differences in the patients, not to the technology. Crossover occurs either when patients in the group offered the technology do not receive it (sometimes called "dilution") or when patients in the control group get the technology (sometimes called "contamination"). Errors in measurement of outcomes can affect a study's results if the technique used to measure outcomes (e.g., claims data, patient interviews, urine tests, blood samples) do not accurately measure the true outcome. Patients can be misclassified as having had the outcome of interest (e.g., death from breast cancer) when in fact they did not, and vice versa. Errors in ascertainment of exposure to the technology can have an effect similar to crossover. A crucial step in a retrospective study is to determine who got the technology of interest and who did not. These measurements frequently rely on old records and fallible memories. Any errors affect the results.

An example of bias to external validity is the existence of differences between the people studied in the experiment and the people about whom you want to draw conclusions (sometimes called a "population bias"). For example, they might be older or sicker. Another example occurs when the technology used in the experiment differs from the technology of interest, because of differences in technique, equipment, provider skill, or changes in the technology since the experiment was performed. This is sometimes called "intensity bias."

Different evaluative methods are vulnerable to different biases. At the risk

TABLE 10.1 Susceptibility of various designs to biases

Design	Internal Validity				External Validity	
	Patient Selection	Crossover	Error in Measurement of Outcomes	Error in Ascertainment of Exposure	Population	Technology
RCT	0	++	+	0	++	++
nonRCT	+	+	+	0	+	+
CCS	++	0	+	+++	0	0
Comparison of clinical series	+++	0	+	0	+	+
Data bases	++	0	++	++	0	0

0 implies minimal vulnerability to a bias.
+++ implies high vulnerability to a bias.
RCT, randomized controlled trials; CCS, case-control studies.

of gross oversimplification, Table 10.1 illustrates the vulnerabilities of different designs to biases. A zero implies that the bias is either nonexistent or likely to be negligible; three plus signs indicate that the bias is likely to be present and to have an important effect on the observed outcome. Methodologists can debate my choices, and there are innumerable conditions and subtle issues that will prevent agreement from ever being reached; the point is not to produce a definitive table of biases, but to convey the general message that all the designs are affected by biases, and the patterns are different for different designs.

For example, a major strength of the randomized controlled trial is that it is virtually free of patient selection biases. Indeed, that is the very purpose of randomization. In contrast, non-randomized controlled trials, case-control studies, and data bases are all subject to patient selection biases. On the other hand, randomized controlled trials are more affected by crossover than the other three designs. All studies are potentially affected by errors in measurement of outcomes, with data bases more vulnerable than most because they are limited to whatever data elements were originally chosen by the designers. Case-control studies are especially vulnerable to misspecification of exposure to the technology, because of their retrospective nature. Data bases can be subject to the same problem, depending on the accuracy with which the data elements were coded.

With respect to external validity, randomized controlled trials are sensitive to population biases, because the recruitment process and admission criteria often result in a narrowly defined set of patient indications. Randomized controlled trials are also vulnerable to concerns that the intensity and quality of care might be different in research settings than in actual practice. The distinction between the "efficacy" of a technology (in research settings) and the "effectiveness" of a technology (in routine practice) reflects this concern. Thus, the results of a trial might not be widely applicable to other patient indications or less controlled settings. Data bases and case-control studies, on the other hand, tend to draw from "real" populations. All designs are susceptible to changes in the technology, but in different ways. Because they are prospective, randomized controlled trials and non-randomized controlled trials are vulnerable to future changes. Because they are retrospective, case-control studies and retrospective analyses of data bases are vulnerable to differences between the present and the past.

Now that we admit that biases are present and potentially important, our problem becomes much more complicated. We can no longer choose the simplest, quickest, and least expensive design. Now the choice must take potential biases into account.

HEURISTICS

It is easy to imagine that this new problem is extremely complicated. In fact, it can be argued that it exceeds the capacity of the unaided human mind. What, then, do we do? After all, this is a real problem that we have been facing for decades.

In response to the complexity of the problem, we have developed a set of mental simplifications, or heuristics, that convert what would be a very complicated set of judgments into a series of rather simple "yes" and "no" questions. The first and most important heuristic deals with the biases. Typically, we simplify our approach to biases by sorting them into two categories. For each design and each bias, we either declare that bias to be acceptable, take the study at face value, and ignore the bias from that point on; or we declare the bias to be unacceptable, and ignore the study from that point on. This said, it is important to understand that different people can have very different ideas about what constitutes an "acceptable" bias. Someone who believes in only the most rigorous randomized controlled trials (what we might call a "strict constructionist") might say the potential biases of data bases (or case-control studies, or non-randomized controlled trials) are too great to accept. On the other hand, a clinical expert might be quite content to take anecdotes and clinical series at face value.

The next heuristic deals with the difficulty of estimating the magnitude of an effect (e.g., the magnitude of the reduction in mortality achieved by breast cancer screening). That can be quite complex, especially if there are multiple studies with different designs and different results. A much simpler approach is to determine if there is any effect at all, without worrying about its actual magnitude. In practice, we calculate the probability that the study would indicate there is an effect when in fact there is not—the statistical significance of the study. If the result is statistically significant, we feel good, even if the actual magnitude of the effect is very small, or if we have not even estimated the actual magnitude.

The third heuristic deals with the difficult balance between the possibility of rejecting a technology that in fact is effective, versus accepting a technology that in fact is not effective. The most visible heuristic is to declare a technology effective when the "p-value"—the chance of accepting an ineffective technology—falls below 5 percent. This heuristic can be applied without ever calculating the chance of the first type of error (rejecting an effective technology). The mesmerizing power of this statistic can be surprising. For years, the p-value of another study that examined breast cancer screening for women younger than age 50 hovered just above the magic threshold of 5 percent. When some authors found a different way to calculate the statistics that pushed the p-value below 0.05 (3), the National Cancer Institute issued a press release that made national news. This behavior is especially touching because almost half the women in the "screened group" did not receive all the scheduled examinations—a bias that overwhelms the meaning of the p-value. But there are other heuristics. Toward the other extreme is the common sentiment among practitioners that unless a technology has been proven not to be effective, it should be considered effective. The point is not that the heuristics are applied uniformly, simply that they are applied widely. The last set of heuristics is the most sweeping. To deal with the complex issues raised by costs and limited resources, we simply ignore costs and limits on resources.

Our main concern is with the first heuristic, in which some biases are declared acceptable and others are not. Consider the implications of different points of view. To insist on seeing randomized controlled trial "proof" of effectiveness before approving a technology, and to not allow case-control studies, non-randomized controlled trials, analysis of data bases, or comparisons of clinical series (call this the "strict constructionist approach") is essentially saying that a patient selection bias is not acceptable (see Table 10.1). However, whenever a randomized controlled trial is taken at face value—for example, the results are analyzed by "intent to treat" without adjusting for crossover—the implication is that crossover, errors in measurement of outcomes, and biases to external validity are either acceptable or somebody else's problems. Ironically, leaving it to decision makers to deal with biases to external validity implies an acceptance of clinical judgment as the preferred method to adjust for those biases.

Now consider the implied set of beliefs at the other end of the spectrum. Those willing to make decisions on the basis of anecdotes and clinical series (let us call them "loose constructionists") are saying either that all the biases that affect those sources of evidence are acceptable, or that it is possible and appropriate to adjust for them subjectively. For example, anyone who draws a conclusion about alternative technologies by comparing separate clinical series of the technologies is either accepting patient section bias and a wide variety of other confounding factors or claiming an ability to adjust for them mentally.

To summarize the main points about biases: Every design is affected by biases. Different designs are affected differently by different biases. And there is no way to escape subjective judgments in dealing with biases. The last point is especially important for what follows. Current evaluative methods rely on subjective judgments for such questions as which technologies require empirical evidence (e.g., drugs, devices, clinical procedures), what types of evidence are acceptable, which outcomes must be demonstrated empirically, when intermediate outcomes are acceptable, which intermediate outcomes to use, which patient indications require empirical evidence, how to extend results to other patient indications, which biases are acceptable, an acceptable α-level for determining statistical significance, and so forth. We can imagine that everything is purely objective, but subjective judgments are all around us. The question is not *whether* we allow the use of subjective judgments, but *how* we use them. Should they be implicit and informal, with every man for himself, or explicit, formal, organized, and open to review?

OPTIONS

Now let us return to the problem of choosing the best evaluative strategy. There are three main options:

1. accept the status quo with its inconsistencies and wide variations in degrees of rigor used by various approaches;

2. determine which of the current approaches is the most desirable, and move the other approaches toward that end of the spectrum. For example, we could make the strict constructionist approach more loose or the loose constructionist approach more strict. Or,

3. develop a new approach that combines the two extremes.

To decide the merits of these three options, it is necessary to return to the objective. It is to speed the acceptance and diffusion of technologies that are worth the costs and deserve priority, and to restrain technologies for which these conditions do not hold. The status quo (option #1) is highly variable in achieving this objective. We suspect that the strict approach is too slow; too expensive; discards some information from designs that, although not "perfect," are at least useful; and inhibits or at least retards the introduction of some effective technologies. On the other hand, we suspect the loose approach is too subjective, too inaccurate, too arbitrary, and too hidden. It provides no information on the magnitudes of the outcomes; the conclusions can depend more on which experts you happen to choose than the merits of the technology; there is no trial, making it impossible to examine the logic of the judgments; and it appears to accept too many technologies that are in fact not effective. Furthermore, the basis for deciding which technologies need which types of evaluations seems arbitrary. Is there really any reason to believe there is something inherent about drugs versus procedures that makes multiple randomized controlled trials necessary for drugs, but clinical series and clinical judgment best for procedures? It is difficult to argue that the status quo is the appropriate choice.

This has implications for the second option, picking one of the extremes and moving everything in that direction. If we believe the strict approach is too rigid, we do not want to move everything in that direction. Would we really want to require 49.5 feet of documentation on every technology, every indication? Similarly, if we believe the loose approach is too loose, we should not trade in the virtues of rigor for it.

The third option is to draw on the strengths of both. This approach, dare we call it the "flexible but firm" approach, might proceed with the following steps.

1. Drop any preconceived conclusions about which experimental designs are acceptable or not, and which types of subjective judgments are acceptable or not.

2. Gather whatever empirical evidence exists, from any design. If a group is in the process of designing a new study to determine the effectiveness of a technology, it is free to explore and submit any designs it chooses.

3. For each study, identify the potential biases.

4. Estimate the magnitudes of each bias (including, when appropriate, the range of uncertainty about the estimates).

At this point we reach the main fork in the road. Traditionally, anyone evaluating evidence would make a judgment at this point about whether the biases are acceptable. If they are deemed unacceptable, the study, and all the information in it, is discarded. If the biases are considered acceptable, the study is admitted and from that time on the biases are assumed to be unimportant. Thus, the traditional choice is whether to take the study at *no* value, or to take it at *face* value.

The flexible but firm approach would take a middle course. It would use formal methods to adjust the results of the studies for biases, and use the adjusted results to make decisions about the merits of the technology. For example, if a randomized controlled trial has crossover, the traditional approach would analyze the data by "intent to treat," which is tantamount to ignoring the bias. The flexible but firm approach would not take the trial at face value but would estimate the proportions of people who crossed over, and adjust for the bias accordingly. If it is thought that patients who crossed over might not be representative of their group (e.g., they might be at higher risk of the outcome), that belief would be quantified and incorporated in the adjustment. Other biases could be addressed in similar fashion. Thus, the remaining steps for the flexible but firm approach are

5. Adjust the results of the studies for biases.
6. Use the adjusted results as the best information available for decisions.

The hallmark of the flexible but firm approach is that it uses formal techniques (e.g., statistical models of biases) to incorporate focused subjective judgments (not global clinical impressions) to adjust (not simply accept or reject) results of studies to achieve the best combination of evidence and judgment. The philosophy behind it is that "one size doesn't fit all." The validity of a particular design depends on the question being asked, the disease, the technology, the results, and the suspected biases, among other things. It is not an immutable property of the design.

AN EXAMPLE

For an example, let us return to the two studies of breast cancer screening in women older than age 50. Suppose we are interested in the effectiveness of breast cancer screening in women age 50 to 64 with a combination of breast physical examinations and mammography delivered every two years (call this the circumstances of interest). The randomized controlled trial is affected by several biases. The main bias to internal validity is that about 20 percent of the group offered screening did not receive it (dilution), and about 5 percent of the control group received screening outside the trial (contamination). Potential biases to external validity are (a) the randomized controlled trial involved only mammography (not breast physical examination and mammography), (b) screening was delivered every three years (not two), and (c) the setting was a randomized controlled trial (not "usual care").

Adjusting for these biases requires estimating the magnitude of each bias. Suppose we estimate that dilution and contamination occurred in the percentages reported (20 percent and 5 percent, respectively), that the lack of breast physical examination and the longer frequency caused the observed results to understate the effectiveness of the combination of breast physical examination and mammography by about 40 percent (with a 95 percent confidence range of 30 percent to 50 percent) (4-7), and that the setting of the trial was natural enough not to affect external validity. Adjustment for these assumptions delivers the estimated effect of breast cancer screening in the circumstances of interest shown in Figure 10.6. The randomized controlled trial taken at face value is included in the figure for comparison (dashed line).

The other study was a case-control study. The main biases to which it is subject are patient selection bias and errors of ascertainment of exposure to screening. The external validity of the study is high because it involved a combination of breast physical examination and mammography delivered every two years in women age 50 to 64 under natural conditions.

The investigators have provided information indicating that when screening was offered, those who chose not to get screened appeared to have an inherently worse prognosis after a cancer was detected (8). Suppose we believe the relative risk of breast cancer death in the women who declined screening, compared with those who accepted screening, was 1.4. Suppose also we believe that the methods for ascertaining who got screened in the seven years prior to the analysis (e.g., chart review, records of screening centers, patient recall, and family recall) were subject to the following error rates.

P("not screened" | screened, cancer)	15%
P("not screened" | screened, no cancer)	5%
P("screened" | not screened, cancer)	5%
P("screened" | not screened, no cancer)	8%

Under this set of beliefs, the probability distribution for the effectiveness of

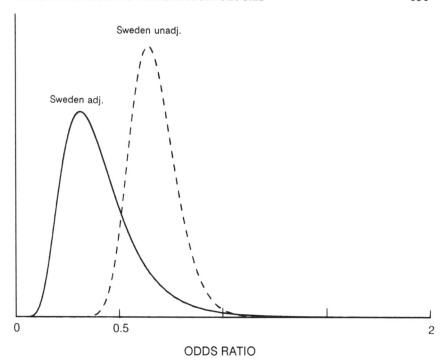

FIGURE 10.6 Probability distributions for Swedish randomized controlled clinical trial taken at face value and adjusted for biases. Face value represented by dashed line, value adjusted for biases (see text) by solid line.

breast cancer screening in the circumstances of interest is shown in Figure 10.7, which includes for comparison the study's results taken at face value, and the two distributions derived from the randomized controlled trial.

This example could be made richer by incorporating uncertainty about any of the estimates of biases, by considering other potential biases that might affect the studies, by introducing and adjusting five other controlled studies of breast cancer screening for this age group (9-13), and by synthesizing the results of all the studies into a single probability distribution.

It is important to understand that the estimation of biases should not be taken lightly. Ideally, bias estimates should be based on empirical evidence (e.g., data on potential biases should be collected during the conduction of a study) and impartial panels should review the assumptions. This example is intended to demonstrate a method, not promote particular numbers. The concept is that it is possible to improve on the current approach, in which data are either accepted at face value, rejected, or adjusted implicitly by pure subjective judgment. It is also important to understand that formal methods of adjusting for biases cannot and should not make every piece of evidence look good. For some studies, by

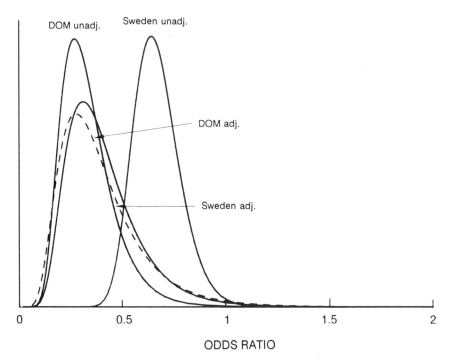

FIGURE 10.7 Probability distributions for Swedish randomized controlled clinical trial taken at face value and adjusted for biases (see text) and for DOM case-control study taken at face value and adjusted for biases (see text). Face value represented by solid line, value adjusted for biases (see text) by solid line.

the time adjustments have been made, with honest descriptions of the ranges of uncertainty, there will be virtually nothing left. The distributions will be virtually flat, providing no information about the effect of the technology.

Many people will be uncomfortable with this example. Discomfort caused by disagreement with the specific adjustments is open for discussion. A panel might be appointed to determine the most reasonable assumptions, and the implications of a range of assumptions can be explored. If the discomfort is due to the attempt to incorporate any judgments at all in the interpretation of an experiment, remember the alternatives. If no explicit adjustments are made, the options are either to accept the study at face value (which violates our belief that it is biased), to reject it outright (which violates our belief that it contains some usable information), or to make the adjustments silently (which is more prone to error and closed to review). If the discomfort is simply because the approach is different, let it sink in for a while.

I can already hear the complaints. From the rigorous side: "What a disaster! Admit the value of subjective judgments?! Tamper with the integrity of a randomized controlled trial by 'adjusting' it?! We've spent decades trying to make the evaluative process completely rigorous and clean—you're undoing decades of hard-fought rigor." From the other side: "Do you realize how much more work this would involve? You want us to wait for experimental evidence and actually describe and defend our beliefs? Don't you realize that medicine is an art, not a science?"

The facts are that even in the strictest forums, subjective judgments already are an integral part of the interpretation of evidence, that the results of experiments already are adjusted, and that the choice of "accept at face value" versus "reject" is the grossest form of adjustment. The current system is not rigorous and clean; it is inconsistent and arbitrary. Remember that under the current system, about three-fourths of technologies go unevaluated by *any* formal means. At the same time, evaluative problems are too complex to be left to judgment alone. Subjective judgments should be used only after all the evidence has been exhausted, they should be highly focused, and they should be integrated with empirical evidence by formal methods.

IMPLICATIONS FOR DECISION MAKERS

The flexible but firm approach will modify the amount of work needed to collect and interpret evidence. For the people who produce the evidence, adoption of a new approach could either decrease or increase the research burden, depending on the current standard that must be met. Compared with the rigorous approach, it should be faster and simpler to gather evidence, because a wider variety of designs can be chosen from, and most of the new options are logistically simpler than the randomized controlled trial. But compared with the loose approach, the proposed approach will require considerably more research, more work to estimate the magnitudes of biases, and more work to perform the adjustments.

The flexible but firm approach will generally make life more difficult for the people who interpret the evidence to make decisions, regardless of whether the current approach is rigorous or subjective. The reason is that in both cases the proposed approach eliminates the "take it or leave it" heuristic that so simplifies the interpretation of biases. It also eliminates use of the p-value to determine when the evidence is sufficient and whether the technology is appropriate (see Figure 10.4). The proposed approach replaces these heuristics with a requirement for explicit identification, estimation, and incorporation of biases. This requires more work, more documentation, and more exposure to criticism.

CONCLUSION

There is no doubt that a change in the evaluative techniques currently used by groups such as the Food and Drug Administration or by clinicians would require major changes in the way we think about medical practices and in the types of evidence required to make decisions. There is also little doubt that we can extract more understanding from existing information, can gather sufficient evidence to make at least some decisions faster and less expensively, and can eliminate or at least narrow the glaring inconsistencies that now exist. The flexible but firm approach would allow us to cut back a bit on the strictness with which some technologies are evaluated, and put more energy into increasing the rigor with which other technologies are evaluated.

REFERENCES

1. Tabar L, Fagerberg CJG, Gad A et al. Reduction in mortality from breast cancer after mass screening with mammography. Lancet 1985;1:829–832.
2. Collette HJA, Rombach JJ, Day NE, DeWaard F. Evaluation of screening for breast cancer in a non-randomised study (The DOM Project) by means of a case-control study. Lancet 1984;1:1224–1226.
3. Chu KC, Smart CR, Tarone RE. Analysis of breast cancer mortality and stage distribution by age for the health insurance plan clinical trial. Journal of the National Cancer Institute 1988;80:1125–1132.
4. Eddy DM. Screening for Cancer: Theory, Analysis and Design. Englewood Cliffs, N.J.: Prentice-Hall, 1980.
5. Bailar JC III. Mammography: A contrary view. Annals of Internal Medicine 1976;84:77–84.
6. Shapiro S. Evidence on screening for breast cancer from a randomized trial. Cancer 1977;39:2772–2782.
7. Shwartz M. An analysis of the benefits of serial screening for breast cancer based upon a mathematical model of the disease. Cancer 1978;51:1550–1564.
8. DeWaard F, Collette HJA, Rombach JJ, Collette C. Breast cancer screening, with particular reference to the concept of "high risk" groups. Breast Cancer Research and Treatment 1988;11:125–132.
9. Shapiro S, Venet W, Strax P et al. Current results of the breast cancer screening randomized trial: The Health Insurance Plan (HIP) of Greater New York Study. In Screening for Breast Cancer. Toronto: Sam Huber Publishing, 1988: chapter 6.
10. Verbeek ALM, Hendriks JHCL, Holland R et al. Mammographic screening and breast cancer mortality: Age-specific effects in Nijmegen Project, 1975–1982. Lancet 1985;1:865–866.
11. Palli D, DelTurco MR, Buiatti E et al. A case-control study of the efficacy of a non-randomized breast cancer screening program in Florence (Italy). International Journal of Cancer 1986;38:501–504.
12. U.K. Trial of Early Detection of Breast Cancer Group. First results on mortality reduction in the U.K. trial of early detection of breast cancer. Lancet 1988;2:411–416.
13. Andersson I, Aspegren K, Janzon L et al. Mammographic screening and mortality from breast cancer: The Malmo Mammographic Screening Trial. British Medical Journal 1988;297:943–948.

11

Attitudinal Factors That Influence the Utilization of Modern Evaluative Methods

KENNETH L. MELMON

This volume has focused on assets and liabilities of data gathering methodologies and the ultimate application of the data to modify use of drugs, devices, and procedures. The medical profession's attitudes may affect the gathering and application of data. The profession's actions seem to reflect a disincentive to data gathering in spite of the fact that doctors and their patients have the most to gain from the acquisition of important outcome information. I believe the profession has unwittingly, yet emphatically, developed and perpetuated a serious deficiency in gathering and assimilating the available data necessary to make optimal medical decisions. The origin of the disincentive and its effects are the subjects of this chapter.

The theme of the conference on which this volume is based contains two assumptions: (1) fundamental understanding of the development of technology will improve effectiveness and efficiency of the development; and (2) the methods of clinical evaluation are key determinants of whether and how new technologies—drugs, devices, or procedures—are developed and applied.

The majority of the conference discussion concerned itself with the methodologies for clinical evaluation that can be used mainly to fulfill the needs of a regulatory process, but secondarily to help in medical decision making. We have not asked whether the regulatory process is sufficient for gathering data necessary for the optimization of medical practice or how attitudes of medicine are pervasive in affecting what methods of clinical evaluation are used or disregarded. I will argue that data generation sufficient for regulation of new chemical entities seems to be the major determinant of the methods of clinical evaluation used and who uses them. Those data are satisfactory for regulatory purposes but fall far short of what is needed to optimize physician decision making on the use of new drugs, devices, or procedures (1-3).

We must clearly separate what is necessary for adequate regulation of new drugs, procedures, and devices from what is necessary for good medical practice. We also must make it clear that the agency of regulation is not legally responsible for the best possible use of an approved device, procedure, or drug. Morally, if not legally, the profession is responsible for the nuances of use that optimize the medical value of new technologies. We should clearly be aware that the Food and Drug Administration (FDA) does not need post-marketing surveillance data (PMS) on drug effects to justify its decisions for release of a drug to the market. Indeed, if the FDA does not need PMS to justify or cross-check the validity of decisions to release drugs, it needs even less information about the post-marketed effects of devices or procedures.

THE FOOD AND DRUG LAW AND CLINICAL EVALUATION

I believe that the Food, Drug, and Cosmetics Act is thoughtful and appropriate. The mandates of the act and the performance of the FDA in relation to the mandates are adequate for their intended purposes. Some will argue that the FDA's actions are inadequate, but few, if any, would suggest greater complications to the process. Should we tamper with the regulatory process so that it collects additional information to ensure optimal use of a drug, a procedure, or a device? I believe that, if we tamper with the regulatory process to meet medical needs, it would so distort the process and focus of regulation that soon it would become impossible for the agency to regulate as effectively as it does today. In fact, some would say that the passive behavior of the profession already has distorted the process and crippled it by asking more than legitimately can be expected from the agency based on the food and drug act.

Because it may not understand them, the medical profession does not seem to have defended the minimal and legitimate regulatory requirements needed for marketing a drug. In the hearings that I have been involved with that examine the regulatory process, I have never heard an individual representing medicine saying, "Senator, despite your responsibility in writing the food and drug act, you misunderstand what we can and should expect from the regulatory process. You even misunderstand what *you* should expect of the process. You condemn regulators for not knowing everything about a marketed drug before it is marketed. Yet to expect more than is known today at the time of marketing may lead to fewer drugs being developed and no better use of those drugs than today."

The regulators are and should be the determinants of the regulatory methods and process in the context of the food and drug act and its amendments. Most scholarly reviews of the process conclude that methods used for clinical evaluation of new chemical entities are quite sufficient for the regulatory responsibilities that have been assigned to the agency. But inherent restrictions within the legislation mean that the process does not include gathering data upon which to base the optimal practice of medicine.

The FDA, by mandate of the food and drug act, works without an explicit definition of safety and efficacy of a new chemical entity. This open-ended expectation translates into the most reasonable and economical strategy for industry to use. The null hypothesis is used to prove or disprove the potential for efficacy of a new chemical. The approval is valid because the method is efficient and the most likely medical use of a new entity cannot be anticipated and therefore cannot be tested for. In a practical sense, one usually considers toxicity the unwanted effects that are found in the process of proving efficacious actions that can be attributed to the chemical entity. Obviously, testing the null hypothesis for efficacy often requires exposure of relatively few patients (usually fewer than 1,000) to a drug and those often for only brief periods.

Thus, it is not surprising that information adequate to prove some of a drug's potential value will not predict the full spectrum of the drug's effects (positive or detrimental) when it is used in the field. The FDA's own studies in 1983 bear out some of the shortcomings of the information about drug toxicity developed during testing for efficacy (see below). While the data are more than sufficient to approve a drug for important efficacy, complete efficacies and the demography of toxicity remain undefined.

A second restriction on the regulatory agency is that it may not interfere with the practice of medicine. This law-based admonition means that the agency in effect has only a binary response to any information obtained about effects of marketed drugs. The agency can allow the whole profession to take it or leave it. That is, the FDA can only totally restrict the drug from the market or leave it on for unrestricted use. The agency usually is not in a position to restrict distribution of the drug, or to restrict use to subsets of practitioners or patients. It should not be in such a position.

Medicine must find the optimal use of a marketed drug while it is being used. Medicine should continue to have this latitude to modulate indications, and put toxicity of marketed drugs into perspective (2,4). We should not be surprised that the vast majority of marketed drugs ultimately are used for unapproved purposes and in unapproved dosages, as IMS America told the Joint Commission on Prescription Drug Use. Because the FDA cannot regulate the optimal use of a drug, there are few incentives for it to search for post-marketed effects of drugs. Nevertheless, that search does uncover important uses for the practice of medicine (nuances of efficacy and toxicity) that usually are less dramatic than would be needed to label the drug as an eminent public health hazard. Only in the latter circumstance is banning truly "legal" or at least justifiable.

Although the FDA may be perceived by medicine as an agency that should help gather data to make therapeutic maneuvers as good as possible, that is not their duty. In fact, to unrestrictedly hand them this task could create important conflicts of interest for them. The agency could then be blamed by politicians for having data that allow initial acceptance of a drug, but later appear to "justify" modulation of medical practice or question established use patterns of the drug. In each instance the agency is restrained from further action by law. Yet if the agency tries to make up for the deficiencies in information used by the profession, the medical officers of the agency become vulnerable to politically driven criticism.

The spokespersons for the medical profession have to begin thinking seriously about the information they want that will be sufficient for the best possible use of marketed drugs. They can start by appreciating the wisdom of the food and drug act and publicly protecting the performance of the agency in its most important legal functions.

Medicine then must develop a clear understanding of the effects that the two restrictions on the food and drug act have as determinants of company strategy used to develop a new chemical entity. Medicine must also come to understand the legitimacy of the restrictions and the responsibility they place on medicine to systematically gather post-marketing data. Medicine must grapple with the fact that the majority of uses of prescription drugs are for unapproved indications. Perhaps that situation is created because the profession is uneducated. But it is more likely that the profession is perceptive and is getting its information on the new uses of drugs from medically based sources that are not interested in or adequate for regulatory purposes. Those sources, by using interventional and observational techniques, can provide legitimate data about how to use a drug, a device, or procedure only after the technique is made generally available.

WHAT IS THE VALUE OF THE EVIDENCE PROVIDED BY PRE-MARKETING AND POST-MARKETING STUDIES?

In pre-marketing studies the manufacturer is simply and legitimately challenged to show a biological effect that is likely to have some medical meaning. In the context of that efficacy, the experiments must show whether the drug is basically safe. Thus, an objective of the experiment is to use the drug for as short a period as possible and in the smallest possible doses in diseases that allow ready measurement of efficacy.

The unexpected effects of a drug, if they are to appear in pre-marketing testing, will have to occur almost every time the drug is given, or at least 1:100 to 1:500 times that the drug is given. To know events that occur as infrequently as 1:10,000 or 1:50,000 exposures can be medically important, but these events can be found only after the drug is used in the practice of medicine (5).

Inevitably there will be legitimate major medical limitations of pre-marketing data for the understanding of a drug once it moves into the field. When the drug is used in patients with a variety of other diseases for which useful therapy is available, and when alternative therapy and devices might be applied to the same indication for which the new drug is used, we cannot predict whether the efficacy expressed in the designed careful studies will be seen. We cannot predict the adversity caused by such drugs in complicated field situations.

When adverse effects occur, we cannot predict whether they occur only in the context of expected efficacy or whether they occur in situations for which the drug was never intended or proven efficacious in the first place. Being able to dissect these kinds of events and to link efficacy with toxicity in the field situation is a key factor in appropriate management of the drug by the profession.

Alvan Feinstein (6) alluded to medical situations in which we cannot fairly or thoroughly test a drug, device, or procedure before it is used in the field. The medical community is the only resource we can call on to verify that the potential efficacy attributed to a pre-market drug actually expresses itself after the drug is marketed. Testing a drug on the fetus would be unconscionable. Many diseases are chronic and slow to respond definitely to any intervention. Therefore, it becomes impractical, if not impossible, to subject patients with these diseases to protracted pre-marketing testing (5). Surrogate endpoints must instead be used to test, for example, for efficacy in the treatment of hypertension and osteoporosis. The legitimate effects of drugs on such diseases often may best be estimated by using the observational techniques this conference has focused on.

Despite the fact that they are not used for regulatory purposes, observational studies complement experimental studies of drug effects. It is impossible to mimic what will happen in the field during the experimental study of a new chemical entity when some type of efficacy is proved or disproved. Observational studies can fill crucial gaps in our understanding of what drugs will do in practice settings, many of which are unavailable for intentional experimental study.

DISINCENTIVES AND INCENTIVES
TO THE GATHERING OF POST-MARKETING DATA

If expectations of pre-marketing studies are legitimate, and if the FDA is truly restricted from interference with the practice of medicine, then the agency has a disincentive to find effects that better serve as modulators of appropriate use than as signals of unbalanced danger. The additional important effects of a drug that make it useful to medicine may actually muddy regulatory waters. Thus, the agency needs to hope that the medical community will worry about itself enough to effectively find the true information about efficacy and toxicity in the field. Those hopes have been answered in the United Kingdom and Scandinavian countries but despite their logic and feasibility have not been systematically applied in the United States. Yet, the most relevant and abundant signals created by drugs, devices, and procedures only occur in our midst and by our orders.

The major disincentives for the FDA to gather more data than is necessary to vouch for defined efficacy with acceptable toxicity stem from the political oversight of the agency. Congressional hearings and the efforts of some public causes over newly found data on drugs can be framed in such a way as to be unfairly demoralizing to the agency. If new and more important efficacy is revealed of a marketed drug, the overseers can ask why it was not found sooner; when serious adverse effects that are not serious enough to be considered imminent public health hazards are revealed, the overseers condemn the regulators for releasing the drug in the first place. Even with such criticism, the agency is not usually able to use the new data to relabel the agent for new indications nor is it empowered to restrict use of the drug unless the information is gathered to meet precise and sometimes unnecessary specifications. Why then should the agency accept responsibility to gather data that would be more useful to medicine (to modulate its behavior with the drug) or to industry (to define the most appropriate market for the drug)?

The law and the restrictions on regulatory action on marketed drugs are foremost in creating disincentives for the FDA to reach out for more information after a drug is approved. The agency has every right to expect academics, organized medicine, or industry to pick up the challenge to get the needed data, because each of those parties generates the data, can easily access it, and has so much more to gain than the agency from getting and understanding the meaning of the data from the field.

Yet each party may have its reasons for wishing to avoid responsibility for gathering and interpreting field data. Academics seem to have unjustly relegated the fields of epidemiology, general health services research, and pharmacoepidemiology to the outer fringes of legitimate scholarship. Industry has been quite suspicious of post-marketing surveillance, probably because they feared additional data would be used in some regulatory or quasi-regulatory manner. Perhaps another industry concern about PMS is that those in industry may not have confidence in the medical value and effects of some of their products. The latter concern certainly could be valid if study were to focus on some of the popular drug-indication pairs that intuitively seem senseless, e.g., the rather widespread uses of B-12 in the absence of real indications or antibiotics for the treatment of viral diseases.

In this day and age of costly and effective drugs, one has to wonder why PMS is not a regular part of industrial developmental strategy to define efficacy and gather data in order to defend against some unjustifiable swipes at entities considered for banning. Conversely, certainly Sterling-Winthrop would have benefited if aspirin's cardiovascular effects were established decades ago. So would it have been valuable for industry and medicine if cyclosporine's effects on Type I diabetes, low-dose heparin's prophylactic actions on pulmonary emboli in hospitalized patients, etc. were known long before today. Only absence of interest retards recognition of additional similar market-expanding and therapy-optimizing data on other drugs.

Organized medicine's lack of effective interest in PMS is difficult to understand. How can medicine restrain itself from pressuring academia and industry to get and use, as soon as possible, the inevitably useful data on medical maneuvers? Sadly the profession has not awakened fully to the value of PMS that will help to optimize the use of chemical entities, diagnostic or therapeutic procedures, and devices. Venning very convincingly pointed out the considerable barrier we have constructed against recognizing and using unexpected signals caused by marketed drugs. As he studied medically substantial adverse drug reactions of the last decade (incidence 1:500 - 1:10,000), he demonstrated how quickly leads on unexpected events caused by newly marketed drugs are found and confirmed but how slowly medicine's habits change to accommodate the new information (7).

Even worse than Venning's observation about our defects in using data about drugs is the way that medicine discovered the amazingly severe adverse responses to practolol. The drug caused three impressive diseases that were not seen spontaneously—complete blindness, recurrent complete small bowel obstruction requiring surgery, and severe pulmonary failure. These diseases were caused by fibrous overgrowth of the cornea, the serosal surface of the bowel, or the interstitial areas of the lung. In spite of the fact that the incidence of these events was 1:500, and that the events were initiated shortly after the therapy, it took several years of hundreds of thousands of courses of treatment per year with practolol before the first case was suspected. Once physicians were told of the first incidence, they rapidly confirmed the observation. But overcoming what seems like the embarrassment of the first suspicion or observation took truly herculean efforts.

These examples show that in spite of many discoveries of important effects of drugs after marketing, the profession does not understand the limitations of the regulatory process and the need to be sensitive and tuned to receive and use those data. Medicine does not seem to understand that possibly the most important information about a drug only will be seen in the process of its use in the field. The profession is not taking advantage of the information that is generated. We are not minimizing the time that it takes to see the event and to transfer the knowledge into clinical action.

The American medical profession has provided very scanty new information about effects of drugs. What we usually do is to simply confirm and report the effects that already have been described. The profession has not shown that it has accepted its role in melding data used for regulatory purposes with PMS information.

CONSEQUENCES OF SHIRKED RESPONSIBILITY BY ACADEMICS AND THE PROFESSION

Politicians readily focus on the regulatory agency's actions. Any open review guarantees publicity and involves little political risk. After all, the public naturally is at least as concerned about safe and efficacious drugs as they are about safe airplanes. But if the medical profession does not describe the limits of the expectations of pre-marketed study of drugs and devices, how can the public? It appears that doctors do not know enough about marketed drugs when they use them, do not press for systematic post-marketing surveillance, and almost never balk at or criticize verbal attacks on the agency and its staff. Thus, the way is cleared for a politician's sharp lance.

The FDA knows the limitations of pre-marketing studies and the futility of extending them to guarantee that all important medical effects of drugs will be known before the drugs are marketed. The agency can and has explained that, in order to find drug effects that occur 1:10,000 times a drug is used in a pre-marketing phase, it requires at least 30,000 instead of the usual 2,000-4,000 subjects for experiments. To get an expected incidence of 1:40,000 with a relative risk of 2 (incidence data in chloramphenicol-induced aplastic anemia), 3,000,000 subjects would have been needed (5). Clearly the profession did not explain what easily could have been expected from it. Few, if any, from our profession stood up for or even behind the FDA to defend the regulatory process when critics said much more should be known about drugs before they are marketed.

When academics and the medical profession shirk responsibility for understanding limitations of the regulatory process and leave post-marketing data gathering to whatever sporadic collection occurs, the pressure on the FDA to know more increases. The agency's expectations of itself for knowing more about drugs and devices than is known after potential efficacy is established is only natural. Yet the drive to learn more runs counter to the legal terms of the food and drug act. The ambivalence these countercurrent drives create probably is responsible for certain irrational behavior of the agency.

Many in industry and some in academia complain that trivial, unnecessary, and time consuming pre-marketing expectations of drug testing frequently add inordinate delays to drug development. This disgruntlement is most likely to occur when the same chemical entity already has been released in a foreign market. Some believe that the delay in release at home is simply to bide time while PMS takes place on foreign soil. By such delay, effects caused by the drug that only can be seen in the field may be revealed. If they occur in the 1:100 to 1:10,000 range and are truly severely adverse, the FDA has in its delay tactics developed a substitute process for lack of systematic PMS in the United States. It simultaneously escapes unjustified but inevitable criticism from political oversight groups that always want the FDA to know more.

The American medical profession has become dependent on monitoring of drugs outside of the United States. Although William Inman is not the only source of information on marketed drugs, it is amazing how much the Western World relies on one man for such vital data. The deficiency of PMS does not simply lead to suboptimal decisions by doctors, it may also contribute to wide-ranging negative effects of technology transfer into the medical field. In spite of the availability of cost-effective and valid methodologies, we can count on the fact that they will not be well applied.

Fewer data than are needed will be gathered to justify and extend the early decisions to market a drug or device or validate the use of a procedure. In a meeting in New Milton, England, in 1986 Ollie Miettinen and Walter Spitzer gathered data that demonstrated that drug banning also is often based on inadequate information (8). The fault for irrational decisions to ban lies not solely with the accusations that a drug may have dangerous properties but also with the absence of organized data that refute or validate that accusation. It was not wrong to be worried about possible hepatic and anaphylactic potential of Xomax and the phocomelia produced by thalidomide. But it was professionally incorrect not to have collected data to balance the decisions. We should have known whether the adverse effects were valid and collected data that demonstrated expected efficacy and potential unanticipated efficacies in very important diseases. If we had been systematic in our data gathering, we would have known today whether Xomax, as opposed to other non-steroidal anti-inflammatory agents, truly could have reduced the incidence of myocardial infarction, pulmonary embolism, and stroke that was attributed to it only after the drug was withdrawn from the market (9). We would have known today whether thalidomide could have a major role as an immunosuppressant. It might have become uniquely useful for some of the most vexing problems in medicine (rheumatoid arthritis, type I diabetes mellitus, multiple sclerosis, lepromatous leprosy, rejection of transplantation, etc.) (10). We have a dearth of safe drugs available for immunosuppression and many transplant patients would have been at no risk for thalidomide's potential to cause birth defects. Unsubstantiated banning can create disincentives and increased risk and cost of technology transfer into our field.

We will never know the true value of Xomax and thalidomide because the signals they were creating in the field have ceased. Are we next going to eliminate coumadin from men with prostatic cancer because we do not want to cause bleeding in patients with myocardial infarction?

The FDA itself contributes evidence of its frustration related to where the line should be drawn on its responsibilities. In 1983, the agency studied the value of pre-marketing studies of 16 recently marketed drugs. The drugs represented 30 percent of the FDA approvals from 1975 to 1981. They were drawn from categories that comprise 40 percent of drug use in the United States. The agency concluded that the average time to the release of the drug was 8.2 years, and that half of the time was spent in Phases I and II. During those phases, relatively little was learned about the efficacy of the chemical, but everything that would be discovered about adverse reactions showed up. No additional adverse reactions were discovered in Phase III when efficacy truly was being tested. Furthermore, the data collected about the quantity of adverse responses exaggerated those that would be found during short-term drug use and underestimated those for the long-term drug use in the field. Not surprisingly, adverse and efficacious effects that followed long-term use were not detected in the pre-marketing tests. To compensate for the deficiency of pre-marketing studies, the agency, probably with tongue in cheek or at least with some frustration, concluded that Phase III studies should be extended. But this conclusion was invalidated by their own data. They had shown that drop-out rates were at least 30 percent if Phase III studies extended beyond 12 to 18 months. Thus, Phase III studies could not be straightforwardly extended into Phase IV. If that was to be done, only the patient group at least risk to continued drug use would be the subjects of Phase IV. What is the FDA to do without careful, systematically executed PMS studies using combinations of the methodologies described in this conference? What can we do about the likely fact that the agency knows the profession does not have but could use better data about the drugs and devices we have at our disposal?

GATHERING BETTER INFORMATION ON USE AND EFFECTIVENESS DOES NOT MEAN CHANGING REGULATORY POLICY

The major factors that lead to overextension of the legitimate efforts of the FDA as they attempt to evaluate the ultimate effects of drugs, devices, and procedures also lead to underutilization of available and useful methodologies. The factors can be summarized succinctly. First, there is no systematic post-marketing surveillance in the largest single marketplace for drugs, devices and procedures. Second, the medical profession has shown little, if any, leadership in developing or using post-marketing signals. The origin of such disinterest probably lies in the misunderstanding by the profession of regulatory responsibilities and the power of pre-marketing testing. We may have developed inappropriate confidence in the sufficiency of the regulatory process for providing data that can be used to optimize medical practice. We certainly have misunderstood by underestimating the profession's role in generating the data we need and relieving the regulatory agency from half-hearted and incomplete post-marketing functions. Finally, because of the fundamental flaws in our expectations of the regulatory groups, medicine has forced compensatory moves that are costly in every sense of the word.

I believe that any serious student (from academia, industry, or government) of the regulatory process has to respect the intent of the food and drug act, the development of the FDA, and the functions and the effect of the process as it responds to the law. The scholar also would have to conclude that what may be adequate for regulatory purposes is inadequate for medical purposes and even for evolving regulatory purposes (self regulatory and/or governmental regulatory purposes) once a drug or device is approved or a procedure appears.

Answers to the problem of adequate data about the use of medical tools must come from the profession. We (the profession) and the industry must back appropriate regulatory decisions. To do this and to generate the ways and means to deploy the methodologies discussed in this meeting we must: (1) understand the value of signals generated by new technologies not only at the time of their initial use but also well through their history. (Where would we be today if aspirin had been banned early in its use because it caused gastrointestinal bleeding?); (2) understand the profession's role in monitoring events and interpreting generated signals; (3) educate ourselves and the government and non-governmental politicians to respect the process and judge it on solid bases that do not employ the temptation to make a drama of science; (4) play a modulatory role to ensure that those who have the courage and sense to use the tools available to them have the wisdom to use them well or optimally; and (5) show the industry not only how to gather and use post-marketing data to help physicians understand how best to use their tools but also to define the market for a product and protect its life so it can be fully utilized.

Criticism should always be available to those who help create opportunity in our environment, but it should not be restricted from self. Applied well, criticism would greatly enhance the efficiency and extent of generation of knowledge and the rate, extent, and use of technology transfer.

REFERENCES

1. United States Congress. Senate. Final Report of the Joint Commission on Prescription Drug Use for the Subcommittee on Health & Scientific Research of the Committee on Labor & Human Resources. U.S. Government Printing Office: Washington, D.C., 1980:1–153.
2. Strom BL, Melmon KL, Miettinen OS. Post marketing studies of drug efficacy: Why? American Journal of Medicine 1985;78:475–480.
3. Snell ES. Postmarketing development of medicine. Pharmacy International February 1986;33–37.
4. Strom BL, Melmon KL, Miettinen OS. Post marketing studies of drug efficacy: How? American Journal of Medicine 1984;77:703–708.
5. Strom BL (ed). Pharmacoepidemiology. New York: Churchill Livingstone, 1989:423.
6. Feinstein A. Remarks made during roundtable discussion. Institute of Medicine conference on "Improving the Translation of Research Findings into Clinical Practice: The Potential and Problems of Modern Methods of Clinical Investigation." May 1989, Washington, D.C.
7. Venning GR. Identification of adverse responses to new drugs. Parts I–III. British Medical Journal 1983;268:199–202, 289–292, 365–368, 458–460.
8. Melmon KL. Adverse effects of drug banning. Journal of Clinical Epidemiology 1989;42(9):921–923
9. Inman WHW, Rawson NSB. Zomepirac and cardiovascular deaths. Lancet 1983;2:908.
10. Mechanisms of reactions in leprosy. Lancet 1972;2:580–581.

Appendix A

Comparing the Development of Drugs, Devices, and Clinical Procedures*

ANNETINE C. GELIJNS

This chapter, initially published as a background document for the workshop discussions that underlie this volume, has three objectives. It provides an initial conceptualization of the medical technology development process within the broader innovation spectrum. It subsequently compares the evaluative strategies currently used in the development of new drugs, medical devices, and clinical procedures. Finally, it considers the implications of these strategies for the rationality and efficiency by which biomedical research findings are translated into clinical practice, and identifies some opportunities for change.

AN INITIAL CONCEPTUALIZATION OF THE DEVELOPMENT PROCESS

One of the essential and perhaps defining characteristics of *Homo sapiens* has always been the development and use of tools, often in response to environmental demands and challenges.[1] In this respect, the development and use of instruments to catch, collect, transport, and prepare food and to make clothing can be traced back to the very origins of human societies. Whereas environmental conditions have influenced the development of specific technologies, it can equally be observed that technology has influenced the human environment, thereby changing its underlying conditions. For example, it has been argued that the efficiency of late paleolithic hunting technology may have caused the disappearance of large animals; the resulting difficulties in finding food stimulated development of the technologies of agriculture (1).

*This paper was partially supported by the Querido Award from the Netherlands Praeventiefonds (Dutch Fund for Disease Prevention).

Throughout history, one can observe this complex interrelationship between the development of technology and the physical, social, and economic environment. For example, making a quantum leap through time from paleolithic tools to the emergence of modern technology during the Enlightenment, the development and large-scale introduction of John Kay's shuttle[2] transformed the textile industry fundamentally and, together with James Watt's steam engine some decades later, was one of the major forces shaping the industrial revolution (2). Since then, technological change has had enormous economic consequences; in modern industrialized societies it has become *the* critical factor in long-term economic growth (3). In addition, it has also contributed to the transformation of social relations, such as patterns of work and leisure, procreation, and communication. But, as Landau and Rosenberg observe, technological change "functions successfully only within a larger social and economic environment that provides incentives and complementary inputs into the innovation process" (4). Both cultural and economic forces (a society's intellectual baggage and tolerance for new ideas, investment in capital formation, savings quotas, etc.), and the government policies reflecting them, have greatly influenced technological development. In comparison to the cybernetical relationship between technological change and environmental factors (going back all the way to the origin of human societies[3]), the relationship between "science" and "the development of technology" is much younger. For many centuries the development of technology was largely based on empirical knowledge arrived at by trial and error and was essentially independent of scientific understanding. However, the nature of technology development has changed considerably over time. A crucial period in the relation between science and technology occurred in the seventeenth and eighteenth centuries, when through the work of such scientists as René Descartes, Francis Bacon, Isaac Newton, and in medicine, Claude Bernard, the concept of nature was changed and the basis of a mechanistic worldview was laid. This new paradigm of the existence of mankind and its world—based on the objectification of nature and the establishment of the experimental investigational method—fueled scientific advances and increased the pace of technological change. In the nineteenth and twentieth centuries, science and technology became truly interdependent, as illustrated by the growth in industrial technology related to scientific advances in such fields as mechanics, electrodynamics, and chemistry (5) and more recently by the rapid expansion in professionally managed institutions for research and development.

This change in the science-technology relationship gave rise to the so-called linear model of technological innovation (see Figure A.1), i.e., results were perceived to flow from basic research to applied research, targeted development,

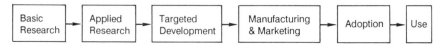

FIGURE A.1 A linear model of the innovation chain.

manufacturing and marketing, adoption, and use. With the rapid expansion in biomedical research since World War II, this model has also become the popular representation of the process by which biomedical research findings are translated into clinical practice. In medicine, this translation process can be categorized into three components: the development of new drugs and biologicals, that of medical devices, and that of clinical procedures.

In other sectors of the economy, this linear-sequential representation has been found to impose a number of important conceptual limitations for the purpose of analyzing the development process. First, it implies that technological innovation is much more systematic than it really is. The stages of the innovative process are highly interactive with many feedback loops. For example, a strong reciprocal relationship exists between research and development: although both scientific and engineering research findings stimulate technology development, the availability of highly advanced technological products and processes stimulates and facilitates research. With regard to medical devices, for instance, the introduction of non-invasive imaging techniques made the central nervous system accessible to direct investigation of the anatomical correlates of function, opening up new vistas for research in neurophysiology. Furthermore, the linkage between research and development exists not only at the beginning of development, but also continues throughout the development process. In principle, the research and development stages are concurrent; for example, to solve problems encountered in the development of a new technology one may revert to the existing body of knowledge as accumulated in research or one may initiate new research (6).

The second limitation of the linear model is that not only research but also the broader environment as expressed through market forces influences each stage of the development process. For years the literature on technological innovation could be divided into "technology or science-push" theories (emphasizing the importance of advances in research and technology as the main impetus to innovation) or "demand-pull" theories (stressing the importance of market demand as the main force in innovation). Mowery and Rosenberg, however, have demonstrated that technological development is an iterative process, in which both an underlying and evolving scientific and engineering knowledge base and market demand interact to achieve a particular innovation (7).

In a general sense, this observation also holds for innovation in medicine, and Figure A.2 depicts the medical technology development process as influenced by both supply and demand factors. Health care technology development can then be defined as a multi-stage process through which a new biological or chemical agent, medical device prototype, or clinical procedure is modified and tested until it is ready for regular production and utilization in the health care market. This development process can be divided into two closely related series of activities: technical modification and refinement (with pharmaceuticals and devices this includes scaling-up for production) and clinical evaluation of a potential innovation[4] (see Figure A.2).

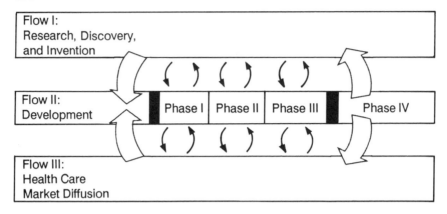

FIGURE A.2 An interactive model of research, development, and diffusion streams.

Whereas it is fairly obvious that current scientific and engineering knowledge (and its accessibility) determines the overall feasibility of specific technological developments, the influence of market demand factors is more difficult to determine. The notion of a "market" in health care is different from the market concept in other sectors of the economy, where in principle the consumer determines what product he or she wants and then subsequently purchases it. The following major differences can be discerned:

• The market demand concept implies autonomous choice and a knowledge of available alternatives by consumers and patients. However, both autonomous choice and a realistic knowledge of the alternatives are often severely limited, and therefore health care professionals usually decide the kind and volume of technological interventions needed (8). In a sense, these professionals are the consumers in the health care market, although their demand is derived from that of patients.

• Furthermore, new medical technologies—in addition to their benefits—nearly always entail a certain element of risk. The beneficial or adverse effects of a medical technology are considered to be quintessentially different from those of many other technologies because, as Renee Fox observes, they affect "basic and transcendent axes of the human condition: life, conception and birth, body and mind, . . . and ultimately mortality and death" (9). During development, the benefits and risks of a new technology are highly uncertain. To reduce this uncertainty, a new technology is subjected to continuous clinical evaluation.

• Finally, health care professionals are usually reimbursed for their services not by patients but by third-party payers. Because patients and professionals traditionally have been insulated from the financial consequences of their decisions, there have been no strong incentives to consider cost in their decision making. In the present-day environment of cost containment this situation is in the process of changing.

These idiosyncrasies of the health care market have prompted government intervention in the development process. Over the years, for example, federal regulatory schemes have evolved to protect the public by allowing only those drugs and devices on the market that are found to be "safe and effective" on the basis of clinical studies.[5] Because individual physicians cannot be expected to evaluate all emerging products, the Food and Drug Administration (FDA) was established to implement the law. In comparison, the development and evaluation of clinical procedures is not federally regulated, but depends heavily on professional self-regulation. Furthermore, because of the government's growing role as a purchaser of health care, government policies have been established to control the adoption of new technologies. In the 1980s the policy focus in this respect has shifted from allocative planning laws, such as the Certificate of Need program, to reimbursement and coverage decision making as important policy tools. These policies are providing strong incentives to evaluate the risks, costs, and benefits of a new technology during its development.

A conceptual framework therefore should also take into account another central characteristic of the development process: the extremely diverse and complex institutional structure within which development decision making takes place.[6] This structure differs to some extent in the case of devices, drugs, and procedures. Researchers in university, government, and industry laboratories provide the knowledge for today's and tomorrow's development process. The development of drugs and devices is largely sponsored by the pharmaceutical, biotechnology, and medical device industries, which have distinctly different structural and behavioral characteristics. The development of devices and drugs takes place both in these industries and in clinical research settings in academia and government, where clinical investigators evaluate the likelihood of benefits and risks in patients. As mentioned, the FDA has an important decision making role during the drug and device development process. In comparison, procedures are both technically developed and clinically evaluated by physicians in clinical practice, most notably those in academic medical centers and university-affiliated hospitals. The broader medical community,[7] consisting both of individual (such as physicians) and of organizational decision makers (e.g., hospitals), decide whether to adopt or acquire a particular medical technology. Patients traditionally have had less decision making power, although this seems to be changing somewhat. Finally, public and private third-party payers, such as the U.S. Health Care Financing Administration, are becoming increasingly important decision makers in the process. In short, the rate and the extent of transfer of a research finding into clinical practice are influenced by the interrelated decisions of a large number of individuals and institutions.

A complex set of social, economic, and organizational factors may affect decision making during development. An instance is the development and introduction of the anti-progesterone RU 486, or mifespristone, by Roussel Uclaf in an ethically and culturally sensitive market (12). In addition to these factors, information on the health outcomes of a new technology influences decision making. As mentioned in Chapter 1, concerns have emerged as to the quality of the clinical evidence that forms the basis for decision making. This appendix will therefore address the following questions:

1. What kinds of clinical evidence play a role in decision making during the development of a potential innovation? What endpoints are assessed during the different stages of development?

2. What are the methods by which these endpoints are assessed during the development of a potential innovation?

3. What are the implications of these evaluative strategies for the effectiveness and efficiency of the process by which research findings are translated into clinical practice?

THE DEVELOPMENT OF DRUGS

The number and kinds of new molecular entities entering development are, to a large extent, a direct result of the activities undertaken and the judgments made in the drug discovery phase. In view of the close relationship between research and development, let us consider some characteristics of drug research and discovery before going into the development process.

Drug Discovery

Although research in various biomedical disciplines relevant to drug discovery takes place in academic, governmental and industrial laboratories, the development process is largely industry sponsored and takes place in industrial divisions and in clinical research settings, often in academic institutions. Historically, close relationships between industry, academia, and government have been crucial to drug discovery and development (13). During the twentieth century the interdependence of industrial, academic, and governmental research has intensified (14,15).[8] On the one hand, industrial laboratories exploit basic biomedical and clinical knowledge accumulated in academic and governmental settings, including the discovery of biologically active compounds (16). On the other hand, basic research findings are also made in industrial laboratories, and the availability of new drugs often permits advances in basic, non-industrial research to be made (17). This reciprocal relationship refutes the popular perception that equates basic research with academia, and subsequently, in a linear fashion, equates applied research and drug development with industry. With the emergence of the biotechnology industry, the reality of this complex interdependence has received new prominence.

Since the origin of the pharmaceutical industry in the nineteenth century, the nature of the drug discovery process has changed substantially. In the second half of this century drug discovery has, to a large extent, moved away from the random screening of thousands of compounds—the prevalent mode of operation in Paul Ehrlich's days—to the more rational design of drugs. This transition was made possible by a burgeoning number of research tools (such as electron microscopes, x-ray crystallography, and molecular modeling), advances in biochemical theory, and an increasing knowledge of physiological processes in health and disease. However, both serendipity and empirical processes of trial and error remain important elements of drug discovery today (18). According to Maxwell (19), four drug discovery approaches can be identified at present:

1. *The basic approach* This approach entails studies to elucidate new biochemical leads or biomedical hypotheses, which may result in the synthesis of new compounds.

2. *Screening of compounds* This screening is usually targeted, i.e., based on a distinct rationale, for instance, blocking of a particular receptor. Because compounds may show unexpected therapeutic activity in other areas, it can also be valuable to perform some general screening.

3. *Molecular modification* Because the first candidate in a therapeutic class is rarely optimal, the objective of molecular modification is to discover improved agents from a "lead compound" with, for instance, a longer duration of action and/or greater selectivity. Maxwell distinguishes between "enlightened opportunism" and "unenlightened opportunism." The former refers to the molecular modification of pharmacological compounds, identified at an early stage of their development, in order to develop an improved agent. The latter refers to making a close chemical variation of a specific drug, which often is already widely diffused on the market. This distinction, however, is not always easy to make (see below), since much of this research seeks to overcome shortcomings of the marketed drug.

4. *Clinical observations* The final source of new drugs can be the clinical observation that a compound, new or old, has unexpected therapeutic actions in patients.[9] That these strategies are not mutually exclusive can be illustrated by the discovery and development of beta-blockers (see Box below).

Over time, the drug discovery and research process has become increasingly complex and sophisticated.[11] Interesting compounds are extensively screened both *in vitro* and *in vivo* for pharmacological and toxicological effects.[12] There has been a rapid increase in the number and kinds of toxicological tests (27,28,29). Following short-term animal tests, long-term animal studies are initiated to detect possible mutagenicity, carcinogenicity, and teratogenicity. These studies often continue for a number of years concurrent with initial human trials. For testing biotechnology-based drugs, however, toxicology studies in animals do not always make sense when the new biologicals are products of human genes and are functionally species specific. More in general, animal tests sometimes have variable relevance for predicting the effects of an agent in humans.

The changes in preclinical testing are reflected in the time spent in this stage of the research process and the costs incurred. While the duration of preclinical

In the late 1940s, clinical research on nerves revealed that the stimulation of one set of nerve pathways, producing epinephrine and norepinephrine, made the heart beat faster and increased the need for oxygen. This research also suggested the existence of two types of receptors in the human body, alpha and beta receptors, that mediate the effects of norepinephrine and epinephrine (21). This work resulted in the hypothesis by Black, one of the 1988 Nobel laureates for physiology or medicine, that blocking one of these receptors would diminish the heart's demand for oxygen, possibly providing relief to angina sufferers. Black and his colleagues at Imperial Chemical Industries (ICI) tried to develop analogues of an earlier discovered compound dichloroisoproterenol (22). This compound had been found to induce beta-adrenergic blockade activity, but also had partial agonist (sympathomimetic) activity. They first developed pronethalol (23), which was found to induce considerable human side effects, such as nausea, vomiting, and light-headedness. They then developed propranolol (24), first marketed as Inderal, which was free of the agonist activity of dichloroisoproterenol and the side effects of pronethalol. The discovery and development of beta-blockers thus demonstrate the importance of the "basic approach" and the interaction with strategies 2 and 3. In the words of the Nobel committee's citation, "while drug development had earlier mainly been built on chemical modification of natural products, they (the laureates) introduced a more rational approach based on the understanding of basic biochemical and physiological processes" (25). Following the introduction of beta-blockers into clinical practice, it was observed that beta-blockers also played a role in lowering blood pressure and preventing heart attack and coronary death. Finally, the proliferation of various beta-blockers has resulted in a number of more selective drugs as well as some so-called "me-too" drugs (26).[10]

(animal) tests was approximately one year in the mid 1960s, it increased to approximately three and a half years in the early 1980s, with a concomitant increase in costs (30,31). Yet, uncertainty remains a crucial element in drug discovery and preclinical research: the attrition rate traditionally has been such that, of roughly each 10,000 compounds synthesized, 1,000 will go into animal research and only 10 will initiate human testing (32).

Drug Development

In the United States, the decision to proceed with the development of a compound, including its clinical evaluation, initially involves a drug company and the FDA. Subsequently it engages clinical investigators, Institutional Review Boards (IRBs), and the research subjects themselves. The 1962 amendments to the Food, Drug, and Cosmetics Act require a sponsor to apply to the FDA for permission to initiate human testing with an Investigational New Drug (IND).

The purpose of such an IND application is to protect human subjects, in part by making sure that the proposed clinical investigations are as efficient as possible to minimize the numbers of patients exposed to the risks of such trials. An IND application must contain essentially all of the information then known (the mean size of an IND is 1,250 pages) on the nature of the new compound, formulation and identification methodologies, stability information, manufacturing methods, the methods and results of preclinical animal studies, the proposed clinical development plan for trials, and the identity and qualifications of clinical investigators.[13]

The FDA classifies IND applications according to a compound's chemical type and its potential benefit, to determine priority for review. In principle, clinical trials can start 30 days after the FDA receives an IND application, unless the agency orders a "clinical hold." After an IND application has been approved, a multi-stage process of clinical investigation starts; the demarcation lines between the various phases are somewhat fluid.

Human testing is initiated with Phase I studies, which ordinarily last between six months and one year. These studies usually involve 20 to 100 healthy human volunteers, except in the case of drugs with potentially high toxicity levels—such as neoplastic or AIDS drugs—where it is considered unethical to subject healthy humans to the risk of these side effects, and thus patients are involved from the beginning. The objective of Phase I studies is to provide information on the dose of an experimental drug that might be used, how often, and especially on potential side effects. While drug absorption, metabolism, excretion, and some effects on tissues and organs are measured, a major concern is acute side effects in humans. Drug administration begins at very low single doses (for instance, one-eighth of the lowest dose that has caused a measurable effect in the most sensitive animal species), followed by multiple doses if no adverse effects are encountered as the dose is increased (35). Safety concerns in this phase may include acute cardiovascular reactions, gastrointestinal disturbances, central nervous system disturbances, bronchopulmonary reactions, and anaphylactic reactions (29). These studies generally involve both laboratory testing and clinical observation.

Development was discontinued during Phase I studies of 20 percent of the drugs that initiated human testing (36).[14] The reasons for these discontinuations are safety (8 percent of the 20 percent), efficacy (6 percent of the 20 percent), and lack of commercial interest (6 percent of the 20 percent). Not uncommonly, chemical and pharmacological research on back-up compounds is pursued in case the compound undergoing development is discontinued due to side effects or lack of efficacy. For example, the anti-arthritic drug, piroxicam, was the third member of a new chemical series (the oxicams), but the first one to make it to the market.

Simultaneous with Phase I clinical studies, technical development activities take place to improve a particular compound's formulation. In developing a suitable tablet or capsule formulation, a number of physical, chemical, and pharmacology issues need to be resolved, such as the use of stabilizing agents (e.g., anti-oxidants), micro-encapsulation, or the development of slow-release forms to achieve the optimum rate of absorption.

Phase II clinical studies involve a few hundred patients and usually take several months to two years. The main emphasis in Phase II studies is to examine the efficacy of a compound in treating the clinical problem for which it is intended.[15] At this point, the endpoints are selected that will be pursued both in Phase II and in Phase III studies. A major issue is the choice of endpoint; should one focus solely on intermediate endpoints, such as changes in biochemical, physiological, and anatomical parameters, or should one also include clinical endpoints, such as effect on mortality, morbidity, or quality of life. These decisions involve complex considerations regarding the disease, the time frame of treatment, and the scientific and regulatory acceptability of the relationship between intermediate endpoints and disease treatment. They can have a considerable impact on the scope of the development process.

Traditionally, a number of intermediate endpoints, such as lowering blood sugar in diabetes or lowering blood pressure in severe hypertension, have been accepted as valid by the various parties involved in drug development. In other, more recent cases involving intermediate endpoints, such as clot lysis in myocardial re-infarction or the increase of hematocrit levels in anemic dialysis patients, there has been considerable disagreement about their value. For instance, in the development of recombinant erythropoietin, a stimulator of red blood cell development, a nine-center, 300-patient efficacy trial demonstrated significant increase of hematocrit levels, while none of the patients developed antibodies to erythropoietin. The FDA found hematocrit increase alone insufficient proof of efficacy and required additional evidence of clinical benefit. The company was able to demonstrate a reduction in the number of transfusions and improvements in exercise tolerance and patient well-being. The license application is being reviewed (38). A number of factors may influence the acceptability of the kind of endpoints to pursue. For example, in hyper-cholesterolemia clinical endpoints such as death from myocardial infarction may take a long time to develop, and thus practical reasons dictate the use of intermediate endpoints such as reduction of low-density lipoprotein-cholesterol. In this case the acceptability of intermediate endpoints is heightened because the association between the intermediate endpoint and the clinical problem is perceived to be strong (39).

The crucial question, however, often is not whether to pursue intermediate or clinical endpoints, but which endpoint should be pursued at which stage in the development process (especially pre- or post-approval). This question is important because the traditional notion of what constitutes valid clinical endpoints is evolving. Since many therapeutic agents for today's chronic degenerative diseases only treat symptoms, the focus in clinical evaluations is shifting toward measuring long-term benefits and risks. Furthermore, it is increasingly apparent that risks and benefits should be measured not only in terms of reducing mortality but also in terms of improving functional status and quality of life. Such quality of life studies are becoming more important in the pharmaceutical area. Recent examples are provided by quality of life evaluations of auranofin and captopril (40).

Phase II studies also attempt to detect short-term side effects. The safety concerns in Phase II and in Phase III studies include cumulative organ toxicity, hypersensitivity reactions, metabolic abnormalities, endocrine disturbances, and if women of childbearing age are involved, teratogenicity (29).

The Food, Drug, and Cosmetics Act requires "substantial evidence . . . of safety and effectiveness . . . consisting of adequate and well-controlled investigations." Most Phase II studies are double-blinded, randomized controlled clinical trials. While placebo control is the design of choice, the agency will accept no-treatment controls, standard treatment, and even historical controls (37). The well-designed randomized controlled trial (RCT) is generally regarded as the statistically most powerful method to determine efficacy (42).[16] The essence of an RCT is that patients are randomly assigned to a treatment group which receives the experimental drug or to a control group which receives a placebo, standard treatment, or no treatment. According to Chalmers (43), a clinical trial is ideally quadruple-blinded: the therapy is disguised to physicians and patients (double-blinded), as are the randomization process and the ongoing results. Both randomization and blinding reduce bias[17]; the differences in health outcome can thus be attributed to the intervention, within the limits of statistical methodology. In a well-designed trial, the numbers of patients and the endpoints are chosen to obtain clinically important and statistically significant results.[18]

The degree of complexity in determining efficacy and safety depends on the therapeutic class to which the experimental drug belongs. At one end of the spectrum are the anti-infectives. Efficacy testing of these compounds is a relatively straightforward assessment of whether the compound kills the microorganism at the site of infection. Due to the acute nature of most infections, there may be less need for chronic toxicity testing. At the other end of the spectrum are psychopharmacological drugs. Determination of efficacy in psychiatric diseases, with a complex interplay of neurobiological, environmental, and psychological factors, is difficult. There are fewer objective tests for psychiatric disorders and one often deals with "soft" measures, making it necessary to subject these drugs to a wider range of tests. As these drugs may often be taken for long periods, chronic toxicity tests are needed. These varying degrees of complexity are reflected in the duration of the development process; for example, the development of psychopharmacological agents takes 3.1 years longer than for cardiovascular drugs, and 7.3 years longer than for anti-infective agents (30).

Within the total clinical development spectrum the highest dropout rate for new molecular entities occurs during Phase II studies when 39 percent are discontinued (36). The FDA analysis lists as reasons for these discontinuations safety (13 percent), efficacy (12 percent) and economic considerations (15 percent). That efficacy and "lack of commercial interest" are prominent reasons for discontinuation is not unexpected if one considers that the main objective of Phase II studies is to determine efficacy, and that the line between "no efficacy" and "not enough efficacy to be competitive" may be quite fluid. With the rising costs of development, studies of the potential market for a drug increasingly occur during Phase II and Phase III studies. The relative prominence of safety as a reason is in part due to the fact that the results of long-term animal studies are usually obtained at this point in the development continuum.

At the end of Phase II studies, a recent change in the U.S. regulatory scheme permits a sponsor to obtain a so-called treatment IND for compounds intended to treat immediately life-threatening diseases.[19] This system makes experimental drugs available at a reasonable cost before marketing approval for terminally ill patients not enrolled in clinical trials. A recent example of a Treatment IND drug is pentostatin, for patients with hairy cell leukemia. With drugs for very serious (but not immediately life-threatening) diseases, a sponsor may request a treatment IND in the course of Phase III studies.

During Phase II and Phase III clinical studies much industrial effort is directed, usually by chemists and engineers, toward process optimalization and 'scaling up' for production.[20] The scaling-up for an efficient production process, involving pilot plant operations and various other process and quality control measures, is a crucial part of the development process.

By the time an investigational drug is ready for Phase III studies, quite a good picture of its safety and efficacy has usually emerged, at least for a market approval decision. Only 5 percent of the compounds initiating Phase III trials are discontinued. These trials commonly involve up to several thousand patients (2,000-3,000), usually are multi-center trials, and are often multinational in scope. On average they last between one and four years. The purpose of these controlled trials and open (uncontrolled) studies is two-fold: to further clarify a compound's therapeutic effects, for example by studying dose levels and schedules in larger patient groups, and to provide information on the side effects and possible toxicity of the drug candidate. These Phase III studies are important in determining what will be in a package insert for the drug, and thus what market claims can be made for a new entity in advertising.

There are inherent limits to how much can be known about a drug prior to its general use in everyday practice. It is well accepted that the detection of delayed or rare (less than 1:10,000) adverse events may require long time periods of exposure, a latent period to have expired, or the exposure of thousands of patients. Wardell et al. (45) point out that a sample size of 306,000 for each group would be needed to detect a difference between an incidence rate of 1/10,000 and 2/10,000 at the 90 percent power level (using a two-sided test, α 0.05). Some serious toxicity may occur much less frequently, for instance chloramphenicol-induced aplastic anemia probably occurs only in 1:40,000 to 1:50,000 exposures (46). However, for side effects of drugs that have less than fatal consequences but are medically important, the important difference to detect is between 1:500 and 1:1,000 or 1:10,000. Furthermore, as Wiener (47) argues, failure to detect adverse effects in Phase III studies may be more than a matter of time and numbers. Side effects may be influenced by environmental factors and variations in physician or patient characteristics (such as differing pharmacogenetic profiles or the use of other drugs, etc.). The occurrence of these side effects may go unnoticed in carefully controlled and selected pre-marketing studies; detection will require actual patient care settings. While the full picture of the risks involved may become apparent only with the widespread diffusion of a drug, an equal argument can be made about benefits. The full range of information on effectiveness of a drug cannot be expected to emerge in Phase III clinical trials that are designed to test the null hypothesis of efficacy. The eligibility criteria for these trials almost invariably excludes a spectrum of at-risk patients, such as those with multi-morbidities, those using many drugs, and special patient groups, such as pregnant women, newborns, children or the very old.[21] Thus, the findings of RCTs may not easily be applicable to the total patient population, especially if linearity cannot be assumed in extrapolation (48). It follows that pre-marketing clinical studies are of necessity incomplete in developing information that can be used to optimize medical use of a drug. A marketing approval decision therefore can never be an all-benefits-known and no-risk situation.[22]

At the end of Phase III trials a New Drug Application (NDA) or, in the case of a biological, a Product License Application is usually submitted to the regulatory agency, with a request for approval to market a specific compound for the indications specified in the application. The FDA ranks NDAs according to their review priority (49).[23] A drug, for instance, that is a "new molecular entity" not previously marketed in the United States and that promises to provide "important therapeutic gain" (i.e., may diagnose or treat a disease not adequately treated or diagnosed by any marketed drug) receives the highest priority rating. An NDA contains detailed information on the laboratory formulation and chemistry of the drug, the results of all investigations, the manufacturing process, quality control procedures, the labeling of the drug, and samples of the drug in its proposed dose and form. Commonly an NDA encompasses over 100 volumes of information containing 60,000 pages each. Electronic NDAs, which contain the data in machine-readable form, are becoming more common and may prove important in facilitating the FDA review process. This review process involves a team consisting of at least a medical officer, a pharmacologist, and a chemist.[24] If applications concern significant new drugs or involve complex issues, they may be referred to an advisory committee for review and recommendations. With regard to biologics, licensing committees are used to provide the expertise as appropriate to the product. The FDA review time takes 2.5 to 3 years on average (30).

Drug Diffusion and Post-Marketing Surveillance

After a new drug is approved for marketing, coverage and reimbursement decisions by third-party payers can affect the diffusion of a drug and hence the development continuum.[25] These decisions should be placed within the context of a country's health care reimbursement policies. At present, these policies are changing in an attempt to contain health care costs; see, for instance, Medicare's prospective payment system, pro-generic substitution laws, and restrictive hospital formularies. With these changes, coverage is becoming a more important decision point in the process, as illustrated by the heated debate surrounding Medicare's decision not to authorize extra reimbursement for tissue plasminogen activator. One consequence is that cost analyses and cost effectiveness studies are becoming a much more prominent part of a drug's evaluation. However, these analyses and their influence on decision making are outside the scope of this paper.[26]

Following the marketing approval decision, a new drug generally diffuses into clinical practice (with the active help of marketing professionals). With the present-day chronic diseases some of the most important therapeutic information, both on rare and delayed side effects and on long-term effectiveness, can be provided only after a new drug has been used in everyday practice. The objective of so-called Phase IV (or post-marketing) studies is to provide this information. This can be done by performing additional controlled clinical trials or by using observational (non-experimental) surveillance systems. The importance of these studies is underlined by the fact that new indications often are discovered only in clinical practice and subsequently drugs may be prescribed for these unapproved indications. One should realize that the FDA only regulates the introduction of new drugs and not their use in medical practice. Only experimental Phase IV studies may be used to request approval for a new indication and to change the drug labeling. In addition, these studies have sometimes been encouraged by manufacturers from a marketing standpoint, to create a pool of physicians familiar with the drug (52).

Most industrialized countries have some kind of post-marketing surveillance system to detect potential adverse effects. Such a system generally depends on a variety of methodological approaches, as no single method is fully effective. One approach depends on adverse effect reporting (53). In the United States, physicians traditionally report suspected adverse effects voluntarily to the company (the Food, Drug, and Cosmetics Act requires manufacturers in turn to immediately report these effects to the FDA). In addition, physicians may voluntarily report suspected adverse effects directly to the regulatory agency, to the medical literature, or to disease or specialty registries.[27] While advantages of adverse effect reporting are its potential coverage of the entire population and low operation costs, important weaknesses are found in incompleteness and inaccuracy. For example, due to a variety of factors, there is considerable under-reporting; the overall return on the U.K. Yellow Card System is estimated to be only 10 percent. With adverse effect reporting one also cannot measure the incidence of the risk. Furthermore, this reporting is by nature a hypothesis-generating activity; the subsequent testing of the hypothesis will depend on other methods.

Methodological approaches for further analysis of the adverse events reported by physicians or manufacturers (and for monitoring signals of suspected adverse effects) include experimental and observational methods. While experimental methods have especially been applied to further examine efficacy post-approval, risk measurements in specific patient populations are sometimes also undertaken. At present, however, there is increasing interest in epidemiological studies, such as case-control and cohort studies, to measure adverse drug effects.[28] The advantage of cohort studies is that they can establish the likely incidence of the risk. Disadvantages are that they are potentially expensive and may yield the results more slowly than case-control studies. Case-control studies are useful if the frequency of events is very rare (up to 1:10,000). Disadvantages are that controls are often difficult to establish and the studies cannot establish absolute risk.

The proliferation of large-scale automated data bases, such as those maintained by health maintenance organizations or Medicaid, may open up exciting opportunities to study a drug under general conditions of use. These data bases may contain demographic data, drug prescription data, or patient hospital admission and discharge data. With advances in computer capabilities it is increasingly possible to link different data bases, for instance, pharmacy records with medical record data bases (55). In essence, the Drug Surveillance Research Unit, initiated by Inman (56) in the United Kingdom in 1980, is based on this principle.[29]

In the same vein, the FDA has carried out a number of hypothesis-testing studies using Medicaid and other medical record linkage data bases. Industry is also increasing its efforts in pharmacoepidemiological research. As these large-scale data bases exist for other reasons, their operating costs are much lower than those associated with registries. In addition, they may lack the reporting bias and the inadequate follow-up that renders case studies problematic (57). However, limitations exist in the adequacy of the data collected in these data bases (see below).

As argued above, Phase IV studies also need to examine the long-term effectiveness of a drug. Since the early 1970s, the FDA has sometimes requested post-approval research as a condition of approval, often with good reason (see, for instance, the approval of levodopa). Studies done post approval to examine the benefits of a drug in different patient populations or with different dosages are usually an extension of the type of studies done before marketing approval (58). In addition a number of large-scale randomized trials have also been undertaken post approval that were funded not by the sponsor but, for instance, by the National Heart, Lung, and Blood Institute. In view of the very high costs associated with these large-scale trials (between $10 million and $100 million), the number of such RCTs is limited (59). Furthermore, as mentioned above, the RCT may not always be most helpful as a foundation for therapeutic decisions.

It has therefore been proposed that modern observational methods could play an important complementary role to the RCT for assessing the effectiveness of a drug. Major weaknesses traditionally associated with these methods have made the determination of the cause-and-effect relationships between drug use and outcomes more difficult.[30] However, in recent years there have been advances in the design and the execution of observational studies, which may address some of these weaknesses.

THE DEVELOPMENT OF MEDICAL DEVICES

Over the past quarter century there has been an acceleration in the development of new medical devices, in part because of rapidly expanding scientific and engineering knowledge (61). In view of the reciprocal relationship between research and development, we will briefly consider the interactions between the research and invention phase of medical devices and the development phase.

The Invention of Medical Devices

In addition to basic biomedical and clinical research, bioengineering research, which builds on advances in the physical sciences, mathematics, and engineering in other sectors, provides an important contribution to the knowledge base underlying medical device development.[31] Basic bioengineering research predominantly takes place in university and government laboratories. In contrast to some European countries and Japan, funding for fundamental research in biomedical engineering is relatively small in the United States (e.g., 1 percent of the National Institutes of Health budget) and is dispersed through a number of agencies (62). Compared with the United States, the Federal Republic of Germany has nearly double the amount of space and equipment for bioengineering research (63). Some recent efforts, however, may ameliorate this situation. The National Science Foundation, for instance, has established a program to fund high-risk fundamental bioengineering research. On the applied research side, the Small Business Innovation Research program was established in the early 1980s by the National Institutes of Health to provide R&D grants or contracts to small businesses. According to an OTA analysis, 40 percent of grant applications in 1983 concerned medical devices and 23 percent of these applications were funded (64).

Federal support is complemented by private investment, especially in applied research. In 1986, the medical device industry invested on average 7.5 percent of sales in R&D (65). In 1979, medical device firms in the five medical device Standard Industrial Classification codes (x-ray and electromedical equipment, surgical and medical instruments, surgical appliances and supplies, dental equipment and supplies, ophthalmic goods) reported that 3.7 percent of their company-sponsored R&D budget was basic research and 23 percent was applied research (64,66).

The investment in research depends on the type of device as well as the kind of firm involved. As Spilker observes, medical devices are a much more heterogenous group of products than drugs in terms of design, use, and purpose; many devices never come in contact with patients, some do briefly, and others do permanently (67). There are roughly 1,700 different types of medical devices and 50,000 separate products (64). Clearly, the research required for the invention of disposable needles is very different from that for the invention of a CT scanner.[32] Equally, there is much more variety in the kinds of firms that invent and develop medical devices than is the case with drugs. The industry is characterized by a large number of small firms; approximately 50 percent of U.S. medical device manufacturers have fewer than 20 employees. Large companies, however, dominate the industry in terms of sales (68). According to Roberts, small firms and even individuals produce most of the innovations in the early stages of developing a new class of medical devices, whereas larger firms play an especially important role later on in the development process (sometimes through the acquisition of small firms). As Roberts put it, the invention of "medical devices is usually based on engineering problem solving by individuals or small firms, is often incremental rather than radical, seldom depends on the results of long-term research in the basic sciences, and generally does not reflect the recent generation of fundamental new knowledge. It is a very different endeavor from drug innovation, indeed" (68). This observation, however, is not as easily applicable to radical innovations, such as those in modern imaging devices, which require large-scale investments in research and development. Such resource-intensive innovations usually take place in large firms.

After a product is invented, a patent application may be filed. While patent protection is extremely important to the pharmaceutical research and development process—partially because of the long duration of the R&D process and the relative ease with which drugs can be copied—the value of patent protection in medical device development is much less evident. In the device area, it probably is easier to invent around a patent, and the research and development time is generally much shorter. Furthermore, with devices that require large capital costs, the need for large-scale investments may prevent competitors from entering the market, and small firms may depend more on trade secrets.

Whereas the potential users of new medical devices, i.e., the physician-researchers, may play an important role during the development process, they also may be crucial to the *invention* of medical device prototypes. Not only do they identify the clinical need for a new device or for improvements in existing devices, but they may also be the innovators and builders of the original prototype. Von Hippel first described the importance of users in the invention of such scientific instruments as gas chromatography, nuclear magnetic resonance, ultraviolet spectrophotometry, and transmission electron microscopy (69). He concluded that 80 percent to 100 percent of the key innovations in these four fields were originated by users and not the ultimate manufacturers. Von Hippel and Finkelstein underlined the importance of users with regard to the automated clinical chemical analyzer (70). For example, the initial prototype of an auto analyzer was developed by Skeggs in the pathology department of Case Western Reserve University; Technicon then made a licensing agreement with Skeggs to patent the auto analyzer and further developed and marketed the machine (71). Shaw, who analyzed 34 medical equipment innovations in Great Britain presented similar results[33] (72). It follows that close interactions between clinicians and industry are important to the development of medical devices.[34] Roberts and Peters, however, found that academicians in the Massachusetts Institute of Technology physics, mechanical engineering, and chemical engineering departments and in two large research laboratories did not readily transfer their ideas for commercial development (74). This finding was repeated in an analysis by Roberts (68) of two major medical centers in the Boston area, although this may change somewhat in the present-day climate, where universities and their medical centers are becoming more market-oriented (75).

These considerations affect industrial decision making. In the pharmaceutical industry, the decision to invest in particular research areas involves "potential demand" for a pharmaceutical as an important criterion. If the user-dominance paradigm of Von Hippel plays an important role in some parts of the medical device industry, manufacturers' decisions will be made later in the R&D continuum. The decision whether to pursue development of a prototype involves both technical and market factors.[35]

Medical Device Development

In most industrialized countries, the development of new medical devices is governed by regulatory schemes, either in the form of standards or extended pharmaceutical laws, which focus mainly on safety. In contrast, the United States has passed a specific law governing the development of medical devices. Prior to the passage of these amendments to the Food, Drug, and Cosmetics Act in 1976, the FDA asked Arthur D. Little consultants to provide insight into the safety and efficacy testing practices of medical device firms (77). This analysis revealed that most devices were tested during their development, but that the extent and nature of clinical evaluation varied considerably among products. In addition, there was considerable variety within product categories. For example, one developer of an artificial knee undertook clinical trials in 200 patients, another performed informal trials with 75, and the third used only 50 patients with no set protocol. Furthermore, in comparison to drug evaluations, the criteria of clinical evaluation may differ with new clinical devices. Criteria more often include user acceptability, either of the design or of the reliability and ease of use in the clinical setting, and the competitive advantages of a new device versus alternative devices. Finally, in most cases evaluations did not include the classical randomized clinical trial, review by Institutional Review Boards (IRBs), or were conducted with patients who signed consent forms.

Because medical devices are a much more heterogeneous group of products than are drugs, it is understandable that some variation in clinical evaluation exists. The existence of considerable variation *within* device categories and the fact that half of the clinical investigations had no formal protocol indicate room for improvement. In addition, the risks associated with some devices, such as certain cardiovascular implants or IUDs, became evident in the 1970s. The Cooper Committee was established to recommend device legislation. It proposed different levels of regulatory control based on the likelihood of risk inherent in specific classes of devices, with more rigorous regulation for devices with higher risk potential. In 1976 the Medical Device Amendments (Public Law 94-295) were passed to ensure that new devices were "safe and effective" before they were marketed (78). These amendments divide medical devices[36] into three classes (80,81).

Approximately 30 percent of all types of medical devices are in *Class I*. Class I devices include such instruments as tongue depressors, which do not support or sustain human life and do not present a potentially unreasonable risk of illness or injury. They are subject to the general controls used before passage of the Medical Device Amendments, such as regulations regarding registration, pre-marketing notification, record keeping, labeling, and Good Manufacturing Practice (GMP) regulations.

About 60 percent of devices are in *Class II*. They may involve some degree of risk and are subject to federally defined performance standards (such as x-ray devices). To date, however, no performance standards have been issued by the FDA, and existing national or international product standards apply.

Finally, all devices that are life supporting or sustaining, that are of substantial importance in preventing impairment of health, or that have a potential for causing risk of injury or illness are in *Class III*. For these, the sponsor needs to demonstrate safety and efficacy before the FDA grants marketing approval. Approximately 10 percent of medical devices are in Class III, such as the artificial heart, DNA probes, or laser angioplasty devices.

According to the law, devices introduced since 1976 are automatically placed in Class III, unless the sponsor successfully petitions the FDA to reclassify it as "substantially equivalent" to a device that was on the market before the amendments took effect. The substantial equivalence provision has provoked uncertainty, as the law did not specify if this equivalence referred to safety and efficacy, or to equivalence of the physical characteristics of a device. FDA regulations issued in 1986 state that devices with *new* intended uses require pre-marketing approval. Post-amendment devices with intended uses *similar* to those of pre-amendment devices may be found to be substantially equivalent only if the new technological features of a device can be shown not to decrease its safety and efficacy (81). This may be demonstrated through descriptive, performance, and even clinical data. This is called a 510(k) submission. If a device is found to be substantially equivalent, the manufacturer may rely on pre-marketing notification. This route to the market is much more expeditious than the pre-market approval route, and the impression is that sponsors will attempt to change the design of devices accordingly. Indeed, a recent GAO report found that roughly 90 percent of medical devices reviewed by FDA were marketed through 510(k) review, while 10 percent underwent the full pre-marketing approval process (82).

To support a marketing approval decision, or in some instances a 510(k) submission, a sponsor is required to conduct clinical studies. Clinical investigations of devices are subject to the two basic elements governing clinical research in general: informed consent and institutional review. In comparison with drugs, however, IRBs play a more important role in device evaluations. They review all clinical device studies, decide if the device poses a "significant risk," and approve clinical studies for their institution.[37] The IRB determines if a device poses a significant risk on the basis of an investigational plan. The plan includes a description of the device, the objectives and duration of the investigation, the investigational protocol, a risk analysis, monitoring procedures, and informed consent materials, and it also identifies all involved IRBs. If a device poses a significant risk, a request for an Investigational Device Exemption (IDE) is submitted to the FDA (83). Such an IDE application contains the investigational plan, information on prior investigations, the manufacturing process, and the amount to be charged for the investigational device. In comparison to the 1,250 pages of an average IND, the average size of an IDE is 150 pages.

After an IDE has been approved clinical investigations can be initiated.[38] Data from a random 10 percent sample of IDEs submitted between 1980 and 1986 indicate that most clinical evaluative studies are concentrated in a few product categories; ophthalmic, cardiovascular, and obstetrics/gynecology products account for nearly 60 percent of all IDE investigations. The range of products requiring an IDE, however, is increasing (84).

In contrast to pharmaceuticals, the final version of a medical device is often not created de novo; instead a device prototype is usually modified technically as a result of initial clinical testing (67). The period of learning necessary before a device can be used properly and efficiently may be longer than with drugs. Therefore, according to Spilker, clinical testing usually first involves an initial pilot stage during which the prototype's design and materials are further developed and tested. The main questions are whether the device produces the postulated effect in humans and whether it seems to be clinically useful. These evaluations usually are based upon non-formal experiments (see below for discussion of the argument to randomize the first patient). In addition to clinical evaluations, this stage also involves technical testing; for example, the electrical and mechanical components of infusion pumps are subject to technical evaluations, and a number of bench tests are performed to determine a pump's accuracy and reliability.

After the technical development has become more or less stabilized, a series of safety and efficacy evaluations of the final "initial" product can be initiated. This decision is sometimes a difficult one, as clinical evaluations usually reflect risks and benefits at a fixed point in time. Too early assessments may not reflect the true risks and benefits of an evolving device and the results of the study may be obsolete before the evaluation is completed, whereas the results of evaluations done too late in the life-cycle may be irrelevant for health care decision makers.

In medical device evaluations, a distinction needs to be made between diagnostic and treatment devices. With the former, it is usually not direct patient benefit, but benefits in terms of clinical utility (i.e., its contribution to further diagnosis or therapy) that are to be evaluated. Fineberg has formulated a hierarchy of criteria for diagnostic technology evaluations: technical capacity, diagnostic accuracy, diagnostic and therapeutic impact, and patient outcomes (85). Generally, evaluations provide information on the technical and diagnostic performance (not the more comprehensive clinical utility or patient outcomes) of a diagnostic device, and possibly on its risks and complications. The main measures of diagnostic performance are sensitivity (ability of a test to detect disease when it is present) and specificity (ability of a test to correctly exclude disease when it is absent).[39] In clinical practice, however, the question of interest is, if the patient has a positive test how likely is he or she to have a specific disease? (86) Therefore two additional measures, the predictive value of a positive test result (i.e., number of true positives/true positives plus false positives) and the predictive value of a negative test result (i.e., number of true negatives/true negatives plus false negatives) play an important role. These measures indicate the likelihood of the presence or absence of a disease in a tested individual from a given population with a particular prevalence of the disease. In order to compare the sensitivity and specificity of two or more diagnostic devices, the receiver operating characteristic (ROC) curve analysis can sometimes be used.[40] However, ROC analyses require simple models and large numbers of cases, and Friedman observes that they are often very difficult to undertake (88). Thus, most diagnostic tests are evaluated only in terms of their technical and diagnostic performance before marketing. Furthermore, according to Schwartz, the range of patients tested may be inadequate, as they usually involve those with advanced disease, and a few young healthy controls (89). A diagnostic test, however, may not perform as well with patients with earlier disease, which indicates the need for more comprehensive evaluations (60). As with drugs, the question here concerns what endpoints should be evaluated in pre-approval and/or post-approval trials.

Traditionally, most device evaluations lack randomized control groups (67). While this may in part be due to less sophistication in clinical research on the part of many device manufacturers, it may also result from inherent characteristics of device development that make the classical RCT more difficult to perform. The statutory standard recognizes this and is less rigorous than with regard to new drugs; i.e., safety and effectiveness information for devices may be provided through "well-controlled scientific studies" or through "valid scientific evidence." The randomized placebo-controlled, double-blind clinical trial, optimally suited to provide pre-marketing efficacy information on drugs and biologicals, indeed has more limitations with new devices. This holds especially for diagnostic but to a certain extent also for treatment devices; for example, a placebo may be unethical (as with heart valve replacements) or certain situations may not be amenable to observing a placebo effect (as when the patient is unconscious or the interaction between patient and device is minimal). Another essential characteristic of RCTs as used in drug evaluations, patient and physician blinding, may also cause more difficulties with devices. However, creative techniques to eliminate bias are emerging. For example, one physician may insert an implant device while another physician evaluates its benefits and risks. Thus if RCTs are possible at this stage their use or that of otherwise well-controlled study designs, such as parallel study designs or crossover designs, should be stimulated. Generally the sample sizes used in these clinical studies are considerably smaller than is the case with drugs. Ophthalmic IDEs, for example, called for an average of 280 patients, while all other IDEs involved about 150 patients (84).

During clinical studies, much industrial effort may be directed towards scaling-up for production. The necessary production capacity may vary widely, ranging from 10 to 100,000 devices a year. Depending on the kind of devices, specific manufacturing requirements may exist, such as the need for sterility or for a certain shelf life. Good Manufacturing Practice regulations[41] govern the manufacturing process in general. International and national standards may also exert an important influence on the manufacturing process, for instance those set by the Association for the Advancement of Medical Instrumentation or the International Electrotechnical Commission (64).

On the basis of the results of clinical investigations, a device may be approved for marketing.[42] In contrast to drug regulation, the device amendments require that advisory committees participate in the pre-marketing approval (PMA) decision for Class III devices (90). In general, the PMA is an individual license to the developer for a particular device. Other developers of similar types of devices need to submit a separate PMA, with adequate clinical data. Data of previously approved PMAs cannot be used, unless they are published and generally accepted by the medical community. This policy protects each manufacturer's investment in the development process, but it also may stimulate the duplication of investigational efforts, including the performance of unnecessary trials. However, the next model of a medical device often differs in materials and/or design, and these differences may affect clinical risks and benefits. Recently proposed amendments to the 1976 medical device legislation would allow the FDA to waive data requirements for PMAs following that of the innovator. Adoption of these amendments could lessen the incentive for innovative R&D.

Device Diffusion and Post-Marketing Surveillance

An important decision point in the course of development concerns the adoption of a new device by physicians and hospitals, which is influenced by a complex set of medical, economic, regulatory, and social factors (11,91). In the 1970s a number of health planning laws, such as Certificate of Need laws and rate regulation, were enacted to control the adoption of "big-ticket" devices. But after a decade some of the drawbacks of such planning laws surfaced, in part because the numbers of new devices expanded beyond the scope of regulation. At the same time, policy attention increasingly turned towards the payment method as an important tool for influencing the adoption and use of devices (8).

Most industrialized countries are moving away from a cost-based, essentially open-ended reimbursement system to a prospective payment system (PPS). This transition has probably been most prominent in the United States with the establishment of Medicare's PPS for hospitals, based on diagnosis-related groups (DRGs). Under PPS hospitals have a strong financial incentive to provide the least resource-intensive treatment. The system promotes a significantly lower level of growth in service intensity than traditionally has been the case, and the recalibration of DRGs is lagging behind changes in medical practice (92). Although the price system is intended to be neutral under PPS, this is not always the case. For example, the lithotriptor was covered as a medical treatment for kidney stones under DRG 323. But this DRG pays only half as much as DRG 308 for the surgical treatment of kidney stones. Thus, although lithotriptors may improve the quality of care and may be cost-effective for some indications, hospitals have less financial incentive to invest in these machines (93,94). Also, because PPS deals only with payments for inpatient hospital care, there is an incentive for hospitals to utilize technologies that are cost-effective over the short term of hospitalization. There is little incentive for hospitals to use technologies which have long-term benefits, even though they may ultimately have a greater impact on the efficiency of the system as a whole. As the existing reimbursement system affects the market for new medical products, changes in this system may exert strong feedback signals to the development process, e.g., it has been observed that medical device manufacturers react to the demand for products that are cost-effective over the short term and neglect R&D projects dealing with products that are cost-effective over the longer run.[43]

With these changes in reimbursement, the coverage decision by the Health Care Financing Administration has become a more important factor in the development process.[44] Traditionally, the coverage decision making process was based on generally subjective evidence provided by medical expert panels; increasingly, however, formal evidence becomes the basis for these decisions (95). This evidence includes safety and efficacy considerations narrowly defined, but there is a tendency to consider the effect of devices on the quality of life of patients (including their preferences for certain outcomes) and their cost-effectiveness. As such, the change in decision making provides an important incentive to undertake evaluative studies after pre-marketing notification or FDA approval.

Phase IV studies include a number of post-marketing surveillance mechanisms to detect adverse device reactions.[45] The FDA maintains a Device Experience Network that receives reports on device hazards from health professionals and manufacturers. Device manufacturers are required to keep records of complaints as part of GMP regulations. On the basis of adverse reaction reports, the FDA may require removal of designated devices from the market or restrict their sale or use. In comparison to drugs, acute injuries are probably more easily associated with a particular device. A major issue, which needs to be examined, is whether the adverse reaction or event is a consequence of the skill of the professional or inadequate maintenance of the device, or can be attributed to a defect in the device itself (96).

In addition to these surveillance mechanisms, a number of epidemiological methods may be used to detect possible risks of device use. As discussed above, the potential of using observational methods for risk detection is increasing. In addition, information on effectiveness is needed; such information can be provided by experimental or observational studies. Because the life cycle of a device is short and next-generation versions of a particular device may emerge relatively quickly (as with diagnostic pregnancy kits, for instance) the applicability of RCTs may be more limited. An advantage of using modern observational data bases is that they represent continuous monitoring of the use of devices in practice and their outcomes. Uncertainty, however, remains as to the strengths and weaknesses of these methods in providing reliable evidence (97).

THE DEVELOPMENT OF CLINICAL PROCEDURES

The last 25 to 30 years have seen rapid advances in basic biomedical research,[46] strengthening the scientific underpinnings for the development of new clinical procedures in the years to come. A clinical procedure can be defined as any practice of a health practitioner that involves a combination of special skills or abilities and may require drugs, devices, or both. As clinical procedures involving *new* drugs or devices, such as laser angioplasty, have been considered above, this section will especially focus on those clinical procedures which are not to a large extent dependent on new health care products but on the technique of the provider performing the procedure. For example, the development of certain surgical procedures (although they may involve the use of scalpels, clamps, and drugs) or psychotherapy.

Clinical Procedure Development and Adoption

The development process of clinical procedures is very different from that of drugs and medical devices. Analytically, the distinction between the development of radical or breakthrough innovations and incremental innovations is useful. Radical innovations frequently arise in academic or academic-associated centers, where physical and professional resources are available and clinical development is stimulated. The development of incremental innovations usually occurs in a much more decentralized fashion, involving numerous physicians refining and modifying an existing procedure in everyday clinical practice.

In contrast to medical device innovation, which requires—as C. P. Snow would say—the bridging of "two cultures" (that of engineers and that of clinical researchers), the distinction between "developers" and "evaluators/users" may be very fine or even non-existent in the development of clinical procedures. Within the hospital those involved in experimental medicine may be physically down the hall from their clinical colleagues, but often they are embodied in the same person. Physicians who treat patients may at the same time be engaged in the development of clinical procedures. This sometimes may lead to difficult conflicts of interest between the therapeutic and investigational role of a physician. As Swazey and Fox (99) observe " . . . their double-edged role causes stress for most physician-investigators. The strains that they experience are intensified by their typically close and continuous relations with the patients who are also their subjects; by colleagues' scientific and ethical judgments of their work; and by a certain vested interest not only in protecting their professional reputations, but also, in advancing them through recognition for being eminently successful with breakthroughs in knowledge or technique."

In spite of the enthusiasm and fascination generated by potentially radical procedures, the initiation of first human application often remains inherently premature (particularly in the absence of a satisfactory animal model) (99). Therefore this transition often is controversial, as recently illustrated by transplants of dopamine-producing cells into the brain region (in need of that specific transmitter) of very severe Parkinson's disease patients. Sladek and Shoulson, in a review of the initial clinical application of this procedure in *Science*, argue strongly that although " . . . the scientific rationale continues to build for neural grafting as a therapy for neurological disease . . . we could benefit from more *patience* than *patients* (100). Fox and Swazey, in their book *The Courage to Fail*, have described the scientific and emotional controversies that may arise during the development of clinical procedures such as kidney dialysis and transplantation. Their work indicates that radical innovations usually are first applied to life-threatening or very serious diseases, which often have no alternative treatment (101). In these cases the considerable uncertainty, and potential risks, associated with the clinical application of the innovative procedure may be considered more acceptable.

Their analysis also indicates that during their development procedures may often be subject to a partial or complete "clinical moratorium," i.e., human use of a still experimental procedure on patients is suspended (99). For example, mitral valve operations have been performed on animals since the turn of this century. The first application to humans occurred in 1923, but a clinical moratorium was invoked in 1928, in part due to the high mortality associated with the procedure. Following a series of drug, device, and surgical advances—such as those in cardiac catherization, anesthetic techniques for intrathoracic surgery, ligation of the patent ductus, and antibiotic drugs, the clinical development of mitral valve surgery was resumed in 1945 (despite initially high mortality rates). Over time, as surgical experience increased and different patient groups were accepted, mortality declined and the technique became established. Comroe and Dripps have equally underlined how the development process of procedures for cardiovascular-pulmonary medicine depended on numerous advances in different areas of science and technology (102).

In contrast to drugs or devices, no formal governmental regulatory system exists for the development and evaluation of clinical procedures. Their development has traditionally been placed in the context of the physician's clinical autonomy and the trust relationship between patients and physicians. Evaluation of these procedures during development therefore depends heavily on professional self-regulation (for instance, through peer review and IRBs).[47] In this respect, the difference between radical and incremental innovations may also be of importance. In the case of incremental innovations, the line between experiment and individualized therapy often is difficult to draw clearly (103), and IRBs are usually not approached to give their approval for the evaluation of slight modifications of existing procedures. This is different regarding radical innovations, and their development and evaluation (at least for those that are federally funded) is generally subject to the approval of IRBs. IRBs, however, do not usually conduct in-depth examinations of the research design (104).

To date, the potential safety, efficacy, and effectiveness of many procedures have not been evaluated systematically during their development. Surgical techniques in the first half of this century were developed by pioneering surgeons on the basis of their intuition and insight, and were tested by trial and error. Many of these procedures attained acceptance in the medical community and resulted over time in useful treatments. A number were discarded, however, often after years of clinical application, such as surgery for constipation. According to Barnes, this pattern of development is due to a number of factors (105). Historically, there was often a poor understanding of disease processes and an uncritical acceptance of established dogma as dictated by leaders in the field. In addition, the analytical underpinnings of clinical investigations, in terms of sample bias, observer objectivity, or standards for adequate follow-up, were often still rather weak. As Bunker et al. conclude in their important work on the costs, risks, and benefits of surgery: "In this respect, surgery shared with other branches of medicine at the time a process for groping for effective therapies, a process that did not have the help of extensive knowledge in the basic biological sciences or the understanding of sophisticated experimental designs to permit logical inductions from multivariate clinical circumstances" (106).

In the second half of this century, rapid advances were made in the methodological underpinnings of clinical investigations. At the end of the 1970s, however, Bunker, Hinkley, and McDermott conclude that surgical development was still often based on inadequate evaluation (107). Examples of procedures that diffused into health care and only later were to be found ineffective for treating certain conditions include prefrontal lobotomies for schizophrenia, colectomies for epilepsy, and more recently, EC/IC bypass surgery to prevent stroke. In a recent article Eddy and Billings provide an extensive argument for the often weak evidence underlying a number of important present-day clinical procedures (108).

The Use of Controlled Clinical Studies

According to Wennberg, many procedures have not received careful feasibility studies during their initial application in humans (109), but have been introduced on the basis of investigations involving historical controls or more anecdotal evidence. Generally, the results of such investigations tend to be more optimistic regarding the benefits of a new procedure (110). On the basis of such optimism and a complex set of sociological, economic, and scientific factors a procedure then may diffuse into more widespread use. Over time, uncertainty regarding the risks and benefits of a procedure, as used in specific patient groups and for various indications, may increase and clinical trials may then be undertaken. At that point in time, however, the acceptance of the trial results has become inherently difficult as an advocate group for a procedure generally has been created.[48]

Chalmers, therefore, has proposed to "randomize the first patient" receiving a new procedure (114).[49] This proposal has not received wide acceptance, because during the initial stage the practitioner's skills and expertise with a procedure still evolve and the risks and benefits associated with the procedure may change considerably. In view of this "learning curve" phenomenon, the initial application of a new procedure will probably need to involve methodologically sound non-formal experimental studies.[50] Such early careful and comprehensive reporting of clinical experience may form the basis for the design of subsequent RCTs, if necessary, or of otherwise well-controlled trials to determine a procedure's efficacy and safety.

The above does raise the question of the timing of these studies; when exactly in the development process should RCTs or otherwise well-controlled studies be undertaken? If an RCT is undertaken too early, the results may be obsolete before the trial is finished. For example, 15 years ago a randomized trial was initiated to compare the Vineberg procedure with medical treatment for coronary artery disease. Two years later the trial was abandoned because the tunnel implant had been replaced by coronary artery bypass grafting (116). If an RCT is delayed, however, a constituency for the procedure may have formed. Bunker et al. therefore suggested the establishment of a reviewing authority to initiate and coordinate such trials as appropriate (106).

With regard to RCTs, one should bear in mind that some real conceptual, practical, and ethical difficulties may exist regarding their use in the development of new clinical procedures (117,118). Double blinding, for instance, is more difficult to achieve. One possible solution may be to have one physician perform the procedure while another evaluates its effects. Controls may include standard accepted surgery or alternative treatments involving drugs or devices; it is generally accepted today that use of sham-operations is unethical.[51] Surgical procedures will also depend much more strongly on the technical skills of the surgeon, who might be better at one type of surgery than another. Van der Linden (27) suggested that patients should be randomized to different surgeons who would perform the surgery they do best. Furthermore, if alternative treatment modalities are being developed with the aim of improving quality of life, while the different interventions are associated with variable risks and benefits, randomization may be considered unethical. As Relman notes, from the patient's point of view, surgical and medical therapy are not simply comparable arms of a clinical trial. They are vastly different treatments with very different personal consequences (113). In these cases, Wennberg has argued that assignment according to patient preferences may be the ethically necessary choice. This would require systematic analysis of how patients value different types of health outcomes (an understanding that today is not yet available) and an in-depth examination of how one will be able to understand the "biases" associated with actual patient choice.

Post-Marketing Surveillance

Finally, as argued above, the full range of information on the effectiveness and safety of a procedure may not emerge in randomized clinical trials, as these trials may exclude a spectrum of at-risk patients. For example, Hlatky et al. (120) compared the patient population in their cardiovascular disease data bank with the patients enrolled in some large RCTs of coronary artery surgery. They found that only 8 percent of their patients met the eligibility criteria for the European Cooperative Surgery Study, 13 percent met the criteria for the large Veterans Administration study, and 4 percent met those for the Coronary Artery Surgery Study. This indicates that the trial results may not always form a sufficient basis for clinical practice decision making.

Therefore, following randomized or otherwise well-controlled efficacy and safety trials, long-term surveillance should be undertaken of the safety and effectiveness of new procedures as they are used in everyday clinical practice. These studies may involve experimental or observational methods. In view of some of the logistical problems involved, it may be especially useful to depend on modern observational methods that enable one to monitor clinical practice and changes in health outcomes. In recent years the use of such observational studies for assessing outcomes of clinical procedures has increased. For example, Wennberg et al. (57) and Roos et al. (121) have used claims data to evaluate health outcomes following prostatectomy, hysterectomy, and cholecystectomy. Given the increased availability of computerized data banks, the possibilities of inexpensive monitoring are appealing. A more extensive examination of the advantages (such as lowered costs, ease of patient follow-up over long periods of time, and the absence of reporting bias) and the disadvantages (such as adequacy of the data for case-severity adjustment and lack of outcome information on quality of life and functional status) is needed.

IMPROVING THE TRANSLATION OF RESEARCH FINDINGS INTO CLINICAL PRACTICE: SOME OPPORTUNITIES FOR CHANGE

The increase in knowledge concerning human health and the mechanisms of disease has been so rapid during the second half of this century that the present era has been described as that of the biological revolution. This biological revolution may prove as decisive for the future of medicine as the industrial revolution was for economic development in the past (122). The extent to which this occurs, however, depends in part on the effectiveness and efficiency of the process by which advances in biomedical research are translated into clinical practice. As indicated earlier, in medicine this translation or the development process includes three components: the development of new drugs, of medical devices, and of clinical procedures.

This paper describes the similarities and differences that exist among the development processes for drugs, medical devices, and clinical procedures. A primary difference concerns the asymmetry of the evaluative strategies employed: over the last quarter century drugs have been subjected to rigorous clinical testing before their introduction into general use, while clinical procedures are still being assessed only in a more *ad hoc* fashion, and new medical device evaluations are to be found somewhere in between. It might be expected that this asymmetry reflects important differences in the effectiveness and efficiency of the three different processes by which research findings are translated into clinical practice. Following are some major observations with regard to these differences, and some inferences as to opportunities for improvement.

The Development of Drugs

In comparison to the medical device industry, the multinational pharmaceutical industry is older, highly regulated, and very research-intensive. The pharmaceutical industry annually invests approximately $6.5 billion in R&D in the United States (about 17 percent of sales[52]), roughly $1.5 billion of which goes to pre-marketing clinical testing. The investments in research, but especially those in development, are consistently increasing (since 1980, an increase of

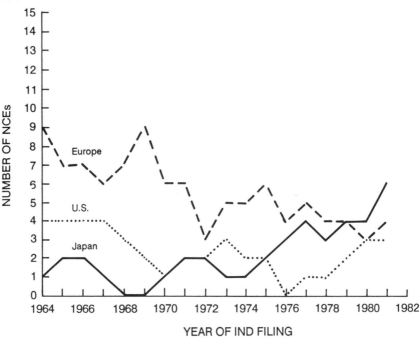

FIGURE A.3 Origin of NCEs on which INDs have been filed by U.S.-owned firms. SOURCE: Mattison N, Trimble AG, Lasagna L. New drug development in the United States, 1963 through 1984. Clinical Pharmacology and Therapeutics 1988;43:290-301.

roughly 30 percent). According to the Wiggins analysis, the R&D process is estimated to now cost $125 million per marketed new chemical entity (NCE) (123).

On the input side, the resource commitments to drug R&D, the relevant scientific knowledge, and the technical capabilities have all grown impressively since the 1950s, but this growth has not been reflected on the output side, at least not quantitatively (124). The number of NCEs entering human testing fell from a mean of 89 a year in the period 1950-1962, to 35 a year in 1963-1972, to 17 a year in the period 1975-1979 (an overall reduction of 81 percent) (30, 31,125). In recent years, IND filings in the United States are increasing again, especially those for biological drugs (126).[53] But these INDs are increasingly acquired from non-U.S. sources. Especially noteworthy is the fact that Japan has been increasing as a source since the early 1970s, by the end of the 1970s surpassing Europe, traditionally a stronghold for producing new chemical compounds (see Figure A.3). A similar trend occurs with regard to the number of new drug approvals.[54]

Over the years these output measures of the development process have been extensively reviewed in the literature and the halls of Congress (see Addendum). The dates given above indicate that the beginning of the decline in the number of new U.S. drug introductions occurred at roughly the same time as the introduction of the 1962 amendments to the Food, Drug, and Cosmetics Act. A substantial body of policy analysis was undertaken to consider the causal effect of these regulatory changes on the declining number of new drug approvals. Originally it was concluded that the decline in drug introductions could be fully attributed to changes in regulatory requirements for evaluative practice during development. Currently, however, in view of the increasing recognition of social, economic, managerial, and political factors as determinants of the decline, it is apparent that no such straightforward link can be established (127). Nonetheless, regulatory requirements—and their interpretation by the regulatory agencies concerned—remain an important factor in the potential rise and fall of new drugs, not to mention the scientific, commercial, and public perceptions of such regulations as determinants of whether and how a drug is developed.

Generally speaking, these regulatory configurations and the resulting clinical evaluations have led to important benefits.[55] Under social and political pressures, these requirements have become increasingly detailed over time. As a result the time-span of pre-marketing development has increased from about 4.5 years in 1964 to 9 years in 1984 (31). This interval has reached a point where access to useful new drugs may be delayed. The tension between increasingly thorough pre-marketing evaluations and early availability becomes urgent in the case of life-threatening disease.

For example, the prominence of AIDS has raised two fundamental issues as to the clinical basis on which decisions are being made. The first concerns the endpoint issue mentioned earlier, i.e., considerable uncertainty exists as to what endpoints should be evaluated during which stage of the development process. For instance, to expand on the AIDS example, the question concerns whether and in which cases intermediate endpoints (instead of survival) should be evaluated in pre-marketing trials. Equally, the question concerns whether and when quality of life endpoints should be built into the developmental evaluation process.

The second issue concerns the balance between pre- and post-marketing evaluation, regarding which some new initiatives have recently materialized. The FDA, for example, has proposed to streamline the drug approval process for life-threatening diseases by shortening the pre-marketing evaluation stage (Phase II and Phase III clinical trials will be merged into more definitive Phase II trials), and by emphasizing more strongly the post-marketing evaluation stage (Phase IV) for providing safety and effectiveness information on a new drug. Even apart from life-threatening diseases, there is a general need for such Phase IV information, because the full range of a drug's risks and benefits will emerge only when it is used in actual circumstances of clinical practice. Drugs, once marketed, are subject to empirical innovation—just like devices or clinical procedures. That is, in the hands of physicians trying to solve problems, new theories are spun out and drugs are used as if those theories were true (e.g., cimetidine). It is only through Phase IV monitoring and surveillance broadly construed (i.e., regarding general use) that the identification of these theories can be accelerated and steps taken to assure their timely testing.

As argued above, the Phase IV studies that would provide this information will depend heavily on observational methods. In recent years, methodological advances (see below) have opened up new opportunities for inexpensively monitoring the use and long-term risks of drugs. These methods may well be useful, not only in providing risk information, but also in providing effectiveness information. So far, however, uncertainty prevails as to the scientific value of the practical application of these methods to medicine in general and drugs in particular. In view of the potential effects of these methods on shifts between "development" phases and the subsequent implications for medical innovation in general, any serious investment strategy for medical technology development must address the possible promise of such an application.

A broader argument exists to carefully consider the potential and problems of post-marketing evaluation.[56] The increasing time-span of development has not only made the process more costly but also has decreased the return on investments by lowering the effective patent life of new pharmaceuticals. The average patent life of NCEs, from date of approval to expiration of the patent, was 16.3 years in 1960 and roughly 9 years in the mid 1980s.[57] The need to consider patent life was recognized in the United States, and the Drug Price Competition and Patent Term Restoration Act was enacted in 1984. The law, however, restores only some of the patent life lost during the regulatory process, as it also allows generic drugs to receive more speedy marketing approval through a system of abbreviated NDAs.[58] The overall result of this law is that the effective exclusive marketing time of innovative products has not increased because generic drugs can be marketed more rapidly. The impact of this law may be considerable since 81 of the most important 100 drugs used currently in the United States will go off patent by 1991, and will thus become generic drugs.[59] Furthermore, the economic climate is becoming much more price competitive, e.g., most states have passed pro-generic substitution laws allowing pharmacists to dispense generic drugs for the brands specified on the prescription forms.[60] Whereas industries other than the pharmaceutical, such as electronics or optics but also the medical device industry, can react to more competitive environments by decreasing the turn-around time of their innovative cycles, such a strategy will be much more difficult in a pharmaceutical industry subject to long and relatively fixed R&D cycles.

Although the pharmaceutical industry has generally been very profitable and recent advances in biomedical research seem to present exciting opportunities for the development of new drugs, the trends visualized in Figure A.4 may constitute an impediment to drug development in the long run. Whereas the effective translation of research findings into clinical practice will require information on the health outcomes of a drug in general use, the above underlines the necessity to provide this information as efficiently as possible.

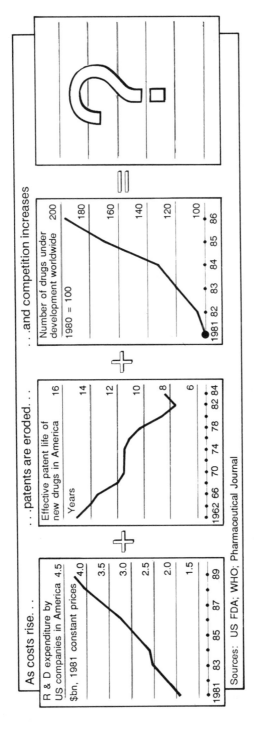

FIGURE A.4 Possible impediments to future drug development. SOURCE: Economist, February 4, 1989:63.

The Development of Medical Devices

Moving from the pharmaceutical to the medical device industry, the latter is younger, more nationally oriented, and characterized by smaller firms; the image of the innovative engineer developing a device prototype in a basement, garage, or study still has some relevance, although it may become a metaphor in the 1990s. In recent years the market for medical devices has been growing rapidly. The overall U.S. medical device market is estimated at over $20 billion dollars in 1987, and parts of that market are expanding at annual rates ranging from 10 to 25 percent (63). Investment in medical devices R&D is smaller than for pharmaceuticals. On average, medical device firms invested 7.5 percent of sales in R&D in 1988 (65), and it appears that this percentage remains relatively stable. Differences in R&D investment can be observed to depend on the size of the firm, and the particular type of device under development. For example, small firms invest almost double the industry average (130).

In comparison with drugs and biologicals, there is a much greater heterogeneity in medical devices in terms of design, purpose, and use, and consequently much more variation in the kind of clinical evaluations undertaken (67). In view of this heterogeneity, the medical device amendments to the Food, Drug, and Cosmetics Act divided devices into three classes and differentiate the level of regulatory control according to the likelihood of risks inherent in a particular device class. Whereas 90 percent of all new medical devices are subject to "general controls" (including good manufacturing practices, pre-marketing notification, and, potentially, technical performance standards), only 10 percent of new medical devices are subject to full pre-marketing review for safety and efficacy (82). It is interesting to observe that, unlike the Drug Act, the device amendments explicitly incorporate in their mandate the need to encourage medical device development.[61]

In contrast to pharmaceutical innovation, there is a steady growth in the number of medical devices entering clinical investigation (84). In the past few years, IDEs[62] include an increasingly broad range of investigational devices. But, since 1980, the proportion of IDE devices that in the first instance successfully completed their developmental evaluation has decreased to 30 percent (although eventually 80 percent are approved). This decrease reflects the more complicated safety and efficacy issues surrounding new investigational devices, a more stringent regulatory climate, and the relative inexperience of many device manufacturers (80 percent of device developers have only submitted one IDE since 1980). In terms of efficiency and effectiveness of development, those who had submitted seven or more IDEs since 1980 had an approval rate twice as high as those who had submitted only one IDE (84). The impression exists that the R&D cycle of incremental device innovations is only two to three years, whereas with radical device innovations (such as ultrasound or magnetic resonance imaging) it is more like 10 years. Development times can then be estimated to range roughly from one year for incremental devices to five years for radical devices.

Unlike drugs, a medical device is generally not created "de novo" but arises in a development process typically representing continuous technical modification and incremental improvement. Clinicians provide significant input by evaluating the clinical efficacy and safety of a device as well as by suggesting technical improvements to enhance its clinical utility. For certain devices the users are also the innovators, designing and building the original prototype (69). Although already fairly common, close interaction between device manufacturers and the clinical community is an even more crucial prerequisite for effective and efficient device innovation than is the case with pharmaceutical innovation.

The initial evaluation stage of a new device usually depends on careful clinical observations based on informal experimental methods. The main question at this stage concerns whether the device prototype has the postulated effect in humans and may be clinically useful. As indicated above, this pilot stage then normally leads to improvements in a device's design and materials. Chalmers (114) has argued for randomizing the first patient who receives a procedure involving a new medical device (or a surgical technique). In view of the technically evolving nature of the device and the fact that investigators usually must be educated and trained in how to operate certain equipment, randomization of the first patient is generally not considered feasible (this equally holds for surgical techniques). This then does raise the question of the timing of (a multicenter stage of) safety and efficacy evaluations, and when exactly in the development process these evaluations should be initiated. If these studies are undertaken too early, the changing characteristics of the device may render the results obsolete. If they are undertaken too late, the results may be unimportant for decision making. Ideally, these studies would be based on randomized controlled trials. However, in many cases, the RCT as generally used in drug studies (involving double blinding and placebo controls) will be much more difficult to undertake, especially with diagnostic devices. In such cases other well-controlled study designs will have to be used to evaluate efficacy. Until recently, however, new device evaluations often are uncontrolled (67), and the use of adequate controls needs to be stimulated. Once the device has been approved and diffuses into more general practice, its long-term safety and effectiveness should remain parameters of the devices's long-term development evaluation. Because device development often involves incremental innovation for a considerable part of its lifespan, and because RCTs are not ideally suited to provide information on a slightly different version of a device, these studies will usually depend on observational methods.

When comparing the rationality and efficiency of device development to drug development and considering the well-known methodological weaknesses of traditional observational methods, it is timely to assess the strengths and weaknesses of new non-experimental methods for providing reliable information about the health effects of new medical devices. In the quest for improved and more reliable methods of clinical device evaluation, however, it is necessary to consider the importance of small device firms in medical device innovation.

One will need to keep in mind the potentially differential impact such requirements could have on small versus large firms in terms of viability, innovation potential, competitiveness, etc.

The Development of Clinical Procedures

As discussed above, the distinction between "developers" and "evaluators/users" is a thin line in the development of clinical procedures. In comparison to drugs and devices, no governmental regulatory system governs their development. The evaluation of developing clinical procedures is based in principle on the trust relationship between physicians and patients. Initiation of development and its evaluation thus depends heavily on professional self-regulation. In this respect the difference between radical and incremental innovations is important. Radical innovations may frequently originate in academia or academic-associated centers, and are generally subject to approval by IRBs. A large part of developmental efforts, however, concern incremental improvements in existing procedures. In cases of incremental improvement the line between experiment and individualized therapy generally is difficult to draw clearly, with the result that IRBs are not usually approached for approval.

There is very little information available on investments in R&D for clinical procedures. It appears, however, that considerable changes may be taking place as to the source of funding in this area. For example, whereas traditionally the development of many procedures was cross-subsidized through patient care revenues, with the changes in hospital reimbursement these funds are decreasing. Very little information is also available on the aggregate number of new procedures being developed as well as on the average time needed for development.

During the development process new clinical procedures generally have not been systematically evaluated in terms of safety, efficacy, and effectiveness. Traditionally, their evaluation during the development process often depended on non-formal evidence or the use of historical controls; this usually leads to more optimistic results as to the potential benefits of a new procedure than would have been the case from well-controlled studies (110). As a result, the scientific evidence normally assumed to support day-to-day clinical practice is not always provided in a systematic and timely fashion. For example, a number of procedures were discarded only following their widespread use, when they were found to be ineffective on the basis of well-controlled studies. For some of these procedures, the weak quality of their clinical evidence is illustrated by considerable geographic variations in their use, such as those for coronary artery surgery, hip replacements, or lower back surgery. To achieve an effective development process for procedures, more systematic and improved evaluative strategies are needed.

Such an improvement will need to take into account that the development of clinical procedures is a very different endeavor from that of drugs and devices. The development of especially incremental innovations often occurs in a decentralized manner, involving change and refinement of a particular procedure by numerous physicians. During the initial development of a new procedure, the skills and experience with a technique continue evolving and the risk/benefit ratio may change considerably. Pilot or feasibility studies at this stage will have to include "systematic and comprehensive collection of clinical experience" to determine whether a procedure works and to differentiate patients according to prognostic factors (107). However, many clinical procedures do not now receive the careful Phase I studies required for drugs (109). If and when the feasibility of a new procedure has been established, randomized clinical trials or otherwise well-controlled studies should be undertaken at selected institutions. The transition from the feasibility study by a few developers to multi-center investigation is more difficult to determine with clinical procedures than is the case with drugs and even devices. Systematic surveillance of early clinical evidence could facilitate the timely implementation of such well-controlled studies. After efficacy has been determined under such trials, evaluation of a procedure's effectiveness and safety should again remain parameters of development evaluation.

Comparing the Outcomes of Drugs, Devices, and Clinical Procedures

Ultimately clinicians and patients, of course, are concerned with choices among a spectrum of alternative diagnostic and treatment technologies and want to know, for a clinical condition, which treatment is best for which patient. The rational assessment of technology thus requires a balanced strategy for assessment that provides comparable information about relevant outcomes for all relevant technological options. This chapter has already noted the present imbalance in regulatory assessment strategies which provide extensive documentation of (at least some) outcomes for drugs compared to other drugs or to placebos, while little attention is given to understanding the relative merits of drugs compared to devices or to clinical procedures. The treatment of angina, gallstones, or prostatism are examples where all three types of technology have been developed, but have not as yet received comprehensive and ongoing evaluation.

This chapter does not intend to imply the need for a federal regulatory system governing the development of procedures. Alternatives to such a system have been proposed. Bunker et al. have suggested the establishment of a central reviewing authority (under which the various IRBs could resort) to initiate and coordinate clinical procedure trials as appropriate (107). The initiation and coordination of studies determining effectiveness and (long-term) safety of a procedure would also be part of such an authority's mandate.

The Bunker model does not, however, call for the systematic comparison of all technological options (including drugs and devices). A more recent model may be found in the assessment teams which have been established by the National Center for Health Services Research (now the Agency for Health Care Research and Policy) to evaluate alternative technological options available in

TABLE A.1 Comparison of rationality/efficiency of technology development

	Drugs	Devices	Clinical Procedures
R&D investment	+++	+	?
Development time	++	+	?
Number of new innovations entering health care	+	++	?
Clinical basis for decision making:			
pre-diffusion	+++	++	+
post-diffusion	+	+	–

the management of clinical conditions. These teams are to undertake the equivalent of Phase I and Early Phase II studies now undertaken for drugs, make recommendations for clinical trials (Phase III), and conduct Phase IV studies for new as well as established clinical procedures. These teams will focus on specific clinical conditions, such as benign hyperplasia of the prostate and stable angina. They will assess all relevant treatments and thus provide information on the relative safety and effectiveness of drugs, devices, and procedures. Drug and device manufacturers could be expected to have interest in helping to fund these teams. Whereas—on the positive side—this scenario would imply that the stronger financial sectors of our health care system would share the financial burden of performing evaluations of clinical procedures, their involvement could result in possible conflicts of interest. This policy question will need to be addressed if the assessment team approach is to prove a realistic mechanism for the systematic evaluation of alternative medical technologies.

In conclusion, serious inconsistencies exist in the evaluation of drugs, devices, and procedures during their development process. The above indicates that these inconsistencies may have contributed to shortcomings in the effectiveness and efficiency by which biomedical research findings and clinical theories are translated into clinical science and useful clinical practice (see Table A.1). Furthermore, these inconsistencies may also have contributed to unnecessary health care costs, if one takes into account that the least systematically evaluated technologies, clinical procedures, are also the most costly.[63] Although these inconsistencies are to a certain extent the result of inherent differences among the development processes of drugs, devices, and procedures, these differences do not seem to preclude a more balanced approach to assessing *all* medical technologies. Such an approach would strengthen the clinical evidence on which development decisions are made, and probably would improve the cost-effective use of health care resources.

This chapter concludes that to achieve a proper balance three issues can be identified that need to be addressed. The *first* issue concerns the criteria or end-points of development evaluation. With regard to determining a technology's safety and efficacy, the role of intermediate endpoints in comparison to mortality, functional status, or quality-of-life endpoints should be clarified. In addition to clinical and scientific considerations, the endpoint issue raises economic concerns; i.e., these decisions may have large consequences for the length and costs of pre-marketing development. Both these considerations would need to be taken into account. Furthermore, following the approval decision for new drugs and devices and the more widespread diffusion of new procedures, it will be increasingly important to include health outcomes in "real world" clinical practice as important evaluative endpoints (n.b. for diagnostic technologies this may be inappropriate). In view of the increasing numbers of alternative or competing technologies being developed, it seems especially important to provide comparative evaluations of the relative safety and effectiveness of technological options available in the management of clinical conditions. Inherent in these evaluations would be the need to incorporate patient preferences for the health benefits and risks associated with alternative technological interventions.

The *second* issue concerns the methods for providing such information. Evaluation of the risks and benefits of new technologies during their development will have to rely not only on experimental methods (including randomized controlled clinical trials), but also on improved observational methods of clinical evaluation. This applies for devices and especially clinical procedures, but also to drugs; for example, these kinds of studies can provide needed information on the long-term health outcomes of drugs in everyday use.

In comparison to RCTs, these observational methods are usually considered to be the weaker methods of clinical evaluation. However, recent methodological advances may have addressed some of these weaknesses. It has been observed that (109):

1. Advances in statistical methods, for instance those in Bayesian statistics, make it possible to assess outcomes for alternative treatment strategies. These methods are useful for assessing outcomes in non-experimental study designs.

2. The increased availability of large-scale automated data systems and improved methods of data base linkage make it possible to inexpensively monitor use and outcomes.

3. Advances have occurred in measuring the effects of a new technology on functional status and the quality of life of patients.

4. Advances in decision analysis provide means to assess the importance of patient preferences and of the uncertainties about the probability for specific health outcomes.

In view of these advances, it seems especially timely to explore the strengths and weaknesses of modern evaluative methods within the wider context of existing methodologies.

Third, depending on their strengths and weaknesses, a policy and an institutional framework will have to be established for assuring the application of nonexperimental methods as appropriate. It is only by addressing these complicated issues that we will be able to improve the effective and efficient transfer of research findings into clinical practice, and thereby strengthen a crucial link in the medical innovation chain.

ADDENDUM

The major decline in the number of new U.S. drug introductions occurred at roughly the same time as the introduction of the 1962 amendments to the Food, Drug, and Cosmetic Act. A substantial body of policy analysis was undertaken to consider the effect of these regulatory changes on the number of new drug approvals. The early literature, however, has some major weaknesses. One of the initial studies by Peltzman (131), for example, indicated that all of the differences in introduction rates between the 1960s and the 1950s could be attributed to the effects of regulation. One major weakness of his model is that it assumes that new drugs are supplied at a constant rate, and therefore changes in supply side factors that would cause the introduction rate to fall are not incorporated. Using a supply side model (a production function approach), Baily subsequently argues that introductions are a function not only of regulation, but also of industry research expenditures and research opportunities (132). He concludes that regulatory requirements have significantly decreased new drug introductions. The measures used to examine the effect of regulation and research opportunities, however, are not very refined.[64] Wiggins (134), in a careful analysis of the subject, subsequently argues that to determine the specific influence of regulatory factors versus non-regulatory factors on the development process one should desegregate the new drug approval data according to therapeutic class. These data indicate that there were changes over time not only in the numbers of INDs filed, but also in the pharmacological types of NCEs entering human testing. If one compares the mid 1960s with the early 1980s, for example, the number of anti-infective and psychopharmacological drugs decreased markedly, while cardiovascular drugs initially decreased somewhat and then increased again, and antineoplastic and gastrointestinal drugs increased steadily.[65] The primary source of the overall decline can be found in psychopharmacological drugs, especially tranquilizers, and in anti-infectives. The question then arises whether these categories were more stringently regulated than other categories. According to Wiggins,[66] it appears that these categories were not regulated more stringently, and thus non-regulatory factors must have also played a major role. Peter Temin specifies the argument as follows (127). He underlines the fact that by far the largest decline can be found in the area of tranquilizer drugs. In addition to non-regulatory factors (such as the strong patents held in this area), he asserts that "the thalidomide tragedy was the proximate cause in the decline, acting quickly through its effects on the direction of drug industry research and more slowly through the governmental regulatory process." In short, this literature does not specify the exact effect of changing regulatory requirements on the decline, but does demonstrate that regulatory requirements are an important factor in determining how, and whether, a drug is developed.

At the same time, a number of studies (41,135,136,137) have approached this issue from a different angle. They have compared the number of drug introductions in the United States with other European countries, most notably the United Kingdom. Their results indicated that on average more NCEs were introduced in, for example, the U.K. market than in the U.S. market. Furthermore, of the drugs introduced to both U.S. and European markets, most drugs were first introduced in Europe. This phenomenon has been described as the "drug lag." Most of these analyses, however, focus on the 1960s and early 1970s, while these differences have diminished since the early 1970s. While the differences in market withdrawals were never anywhere near so marked as those of new drug introductions, the withdrawal rates also converged over time. For example, between 1964 and 1983, eight drugs in the United Kingdom and five in the United States were discontinued due to safety reasons, while after 1974 the discontinuations in both countries are similar (138,139).

Although international regulatory differences thus seem to diminish, a recent analysis by Berlin and Jonsson demonstrates that the Scandinavian countries and the United States are among the more stringent regulatory approval systems, both in terms of the length of the review times as well as in dates of marketing approval (140).

NOTES

1. The characterization of a human being as a tool-making animal should be qualified. Animal species have been found to use a wide variety of tools, although as far as we know no animal species exists capable of handling fire—in essence one of the first human technologies—to its own benefit. A fine distinction between human beings and animals in this respect may be the human ability to use tools to make tools, and to communicate from one human to another the knowledge of how to develop them.

2. Kay's "flying shuttle" in the textile industries was one of the early instances of a machine replacing human labor with technological labor and introduction of the economic concept of work-without-workers.

3. Rosenberg: "In a fundamental sense, the history of technical progress is inseparable from the history of civilization itself, dealing as it does with human efforts to raise productivity under an extremely diverse range of environmental conditions" (3).

4. Within the development process, clinical investigation is essentially initiated with the first testing of a potential innovation in humans. In the development process of drugs and biologics these initial studies in humans have been designated Phase I studies, which are generally followed by Phase II and Phase III clinical studies before a drug or biological can be marketed. Phase IV studies, conducted after an innovation diffuses into more widespread use, may reveal important information

on the (cost-) effectiveness and (long-term) safety of an innovation, which subsequently may be an important impetus for further developmental activities. In this paper we will also apply the terms Phase I to Phase IV clinical studies to the development of devices and clinical procedures.

5. The federal Food, Drug, and Cosmetics (FD&C) Act of 1938, which provided for the premarket clearance of new drugs to ensure their safety, in its amended form still governs drug development today. In comparison, biologicals are governed by a separate law, the Public Health Service Act of 1944. Major changes to the FD&C act were provided by the 1962 Kefauver-Harris amendments, which increased the role of the Center for Drugs and Biologics of the FDA in the development process. The medical device amendments were enacted in 1976 and are implemented by the Center for Devices and Radiological Health.

6. Nelson and Winter have developed a theoretical structure, incorporating both "uncertainty" and "institutional structure" as essential elements of technology development (10).

7. The decision making processes for individual or organizational adopters of technological innovations vary greatly (11).

8. A powerful incentive for industrial collaboration with federal laboratories, such as the National Institutes of Health, in R&D projects was provided by the federal Technology Transfer Act of 1986.

9. The following examples would come under this category: "all the main classes of psychotherapeutic drugs (tranquilizers and anti-depressants); thiazide drugs for diabetes insipidus; anti-Parkinson action of amantadine; anti-inflammatory action of steroids and phenylbutazone; anti-gout action of allopurinol; anti-arrhythmic action of phenytoin and lidocaine; uricosuric action of probenecid; acetazolamide for glaucoma and epilepsy; diazepam for status epilepticus; protective effects of beta-blockers (and the probable protective effects of platelet modulators, including aspirin) against myocardial infarction and coronary death; use of aspirin and sulfinpyrazone in preventing stroke; non surgical closure of patent ductus arteriosus in premature babies by indomethacin" (20).

10. One caution needs to be made in this respect. As the research and development process is so lengthy, a number of companies may start working on a clinical problem at roughly the same time, but reach the market at somewhat different times. Regarding beta-blockers, for instance, the British ICI and the Swedish Astra started at roughly the same time, but ICI was first to market. Astra's subsequent beta-blocker can not be simply defined as a me-too drug.

11. Drug discovery and preclinical research is governed directly by federal Good Laboratory Practices regulations; however, the investigational new drug regulations exert strong feedback pressures on how research is undertaken, especially toxicological research.

12. Patent protection is extremely important to drug research. Usually patents are filed early in the research process, preferably when there is a clear distinction between the active and inactive compounds. There are three types of patents: of a compound; of the use of a compound for a specific purpose; and of procedural methods of manufacture.

13. Part 312, Title 21, the Code of Federal Regulations specifies the procedures surrounding a "Notice of Claimed Investigational Exemption for a New Drug." Over the years the IND regulations have continuously been revised, resulting in a

very complex system of requirements. Concerns were put forward that the interpretation of these regulations was unduly delaying the drug development process. An attempt was therefore made to rewrite these regulations in 1987, but according to the former legal counsel of the FDA this rewrite did not result in any significant changes (33,34).

14. This FDA study (36) analyzed a cohort of 172 new chemical entities that underwent human testing from 1976 through 1978. Not unexpectedly, new molecular entities developed outside the United States are less likely to be discontinued than U.S.-developed ones (14 percent versus 24 percent), as the foreign-developed entities usually have already been clinically tested outside the United States.

15. One of the major changes embodied in the 1962 amendments was to include the provision that a sponsor needs to provide "substantial evidence" of "effectiveness" as well as of "safety" (federal Food, Drug, and Cosmetics Act, as amended, Sec. 505 (d)). While effectiveness refers to the probability of benefits under *average* conditions of use, efficacy refers to this under *ideal* conditions of use. The law uses the term effectiveness to make explicit that drugs are approved and labeled for use under the general conditions of medical practice, not the more idealized conditions often found in an investigational setting (37). Extending this argument, it is for this very reason that we will use the term efficacy in the context of pre-marketing clinical investigations.

16. There are a number of design variations, such as crossover, stratified, matched, and factorial designs (41).

17. Randomization reduces selection and blinding reduces observer bias.

18. For example, the size should be such as to avoid both Type I errors (the likelihood that an observed difference is due to chance) and Type II errors (the chance that a difference of interest is missed due to too few patients).

19. The agency already had some experience with such an approach. For instance, since the mid 1970s promising anti-cancer drugs (so-called group C cancer drugs) were distributed on a limited basis prior to approval through the National Cancer Institute (44).

20. The process by which a compound is initially synthesized, and milligrams to grams of materials are made at the laboratory bench, is not only quantitatively but also qualitatively different from the large-scale production process. For instance, laboratory chemists may use reagents in preparing small quantities of a compound that cannot be used in a large-scale production setting, which may need to produce a ton of a particular compound per year.

21. Increasingly, if a drug is intended for extensive use in a particular population such as the elderly, it is studied in that specific population.

22. Unless, of course, one is willing to delay the marketing of new drugs for extremely long periods of time. This, however, would increase another kind of risk, i.e., the risk of not having a new or improved drug available on the market.

23. The following classification of INDs, and also of New Drug Applications, exists according to chemical type: (1) a new molecular entity not marketed before in the United States; (two) a new derivative from an active ingredient already marketed; (3) a new formulation of a drug already on the market; (4) a new combination of two or more compounds; (5) a duplicate of an already marketed drug; and (6) a new indication of use for an existing drug. With regard to the potential benefit, the following distinction is made: (A) "important gain," i.e., may effectively

treat or diagnose a disease not adequately diagnosed or treated by any marketed drug; (B) "modest gain," i.e., offers modest but real advantage over existing products; (C) "little or no gain," i.e., essentially offers therapeutic benefit similar to that of an already marketed drug. *Orphan drugs,* i.e., drugs developed for rare diseases (in principle with less than 200,000 American patients) are handled under a different system, which explicitly incorporates marketing and tax advantages for the sponsor. Such systems also exist in other regulatory schemes, e.g., the "fast track" system within the U.K. Committee on the Safety of Medicines.

24. The chemist in the team, among other things, requests that an inspection report be made to ensure that the sponsor adheres to good manufacturing practices (50).

25. At this point a firm also needs to determine its price. The pricing mechanisms and the subsequent drug prices, as well as the health insurance or social security schemes, differ considerably by country. In the United States, there are few government restrictions on setting drug prices. In Britain, however, the prices of drugs are controlled under the Price and Profit Regulation Scheme. Under this scheme, the government and the specific pharmaceutical industry agree upon a reasonable rate of return. This scheme thus institutes a target rate of return (in essence controlling profits), and only allows price increases to work through new products, thus providing an incentive for innovation (51).

26. One development deserves mentioning as it directly influences drug development. In view of rising health care costs, third-party payers are sometimes refusing to reimburse even the routine costs of medical care associated with clinical trials of experimental drugs.

27. In the United Kingdom, for example, the well-established system of physician reporting to the Committee on the Safety of Medicines operates through the so-called Yellow Card System.

28. Cohort studies compare people exposed to a drug with those unexposed, and analyze differences in adverse events between both groups. Case-control studies compare groups exhibiting a particular event with those not exhibiting this event, and then they examine differences in exposure to a particular drug. See the Report of the Joint Commission on Prescription Drug Use for an extensive discussion of these methods (54).

29. The DSRU system system has become a second national scheme to detect adverse drug reactions greater than 1 in 10,000, and to evaluate the balance of risks and benefits of a drug. Using prescription-based cohorts as a starting point, this system actively solicits responses from physicians. The response rate is 70 percent, approximately 22,000 general practitioners report regularly, and the system catches nearly 50 million people. Monitored events are followed up by analysis of the medical records of the patients.

30. For example, the series of cases has been found to be subject to different kinds of physician and patient bias. Cohort studies, for example, may include limitations such as the exact specification of the cohorts, the quality of the data in terms of reproducibility and validity, the difficulty of analyzing the attributable agents, and the occurrence of detection bias. The U.S. Surgeon General's first report on smoking listed five supporting criteria to establish a cause-effect relationship: consistency of the association; temporal relationship between cause and effect; coherence with existing insights; specificity of the relationship; and strength of the association. See also Feinstein (60).

31. Bioengineering research will be defined as the application of engineering knowledge and concepts to the understanding of the human body and its interactions with machines, and to the development of new and improved medical devices. This definition is very similar to a definition provided in a recent National Research Council report (62), except that the scaling-up and production of new products derived from advances in biology (i.e., the engineering aspects of biotechnology) are excluded. Those aspects of engineering are discussed in the previous section.

32. In view of the heterogeneity of medical devices, the type of device determines if animal research will be undertaken before a device prototype is evaluated in humans.

33. Shaw found that half of the initial prototypes were produced by users.

34. Allen (73) established the importance of intra-organizational (e.g., between R&D and manufacturing divisions) and inter-organizational communication for R&D performance.

35. With regard to the latter, a recent analysis of the development of devices demonstrated that half of the device firms considered used a formal financial analysis of the expected returns on investment or at least some form of market survey. Many firms, however, relied on informal decision making processes, usually based on a firm's experience in the market for the product (76).

36. According to Kennedy (79), the term medical devices includes all of the items readily identified as devices as well as *in vitro* diagnostic devices used in clinical laboratories and some products previously regulated by the FDA Bureau of Drugs, such as IUDs, or by the Bureau of Biologics, such as arterial grafts.

37. A "significant risk" device is legally defined as an implant and presents a potential for serious risk to the health and safety or welfare of a subject; is purported or represented to be for use in supporting or sustaining human life and presents a potential for serious risk to the health and safety or welfare of a subject; is for use of substantial importance in diagnosing, curing, mitigating, or treating disease and presents a potential for serious risk to the health and safety or welfare of a subject; or otherwise presents a potential for serious risk.

38. In some cases an IDE application is not necessary but clinical trials are conducted.

39. Determining technical performance involves replicability and reliability as important criteria.

40. The ROC analysis allows one to compare the technical performance of diagnostic tests over a range of different cutoff points or reference values that denote a positive test result. This test displays the true positive ratios and the false positive ratios for these different cutoff points. See McNeil et al. (87).

41. One needs to distinguish between critical and non-critical devices. Most rigorous GMP regulations apply only to critical devices.

42. On average the FDA takes a year to approve a PMA (81).

43. As mentioned before, the economic environment in general and cost analyses of devices in particular are outside the scope of this paper.

44. The statutory provision indicates that this decision should be based on whether a device is considered "reasonable and necessary," which has been translated to mean "accepted by the medical community as a safe and efficacious treatment for a particular condition." Based on 13 technologies that completed the full

Medicare coverage process (including technology assessments by the Office for Health Technology Assessment) from the 1983-1988 period, it took 2.4 years from the time that HCFA received the initial inquiry to the final disposition date.

45. A condition of the approval for new Class III devices is that information received by manufacturers on device defects or adverse reactions should be reported to the FDA within 10 days.

46. In absolute terms, the United States invests heavily in biomedical research and development. Shepard and Durch (98), for example, indicate that the United States accounts for 45 percent of funds spent in the Organization for Economic Cooperation and Development countries, and the top five countries—United States, Japan, The Federal Republic of Germany, France, The United Kingdom—account for 84 percent of all biomedical R&D expenditures. If considering *per capita* spending, however, Switzerland and Sweden head the list.

47. It is within this context that medical societies are increasingly issuing guidelines regarding the use of a particular new procedure; however, usually these guidelines emerge after a new procedure has already diffused more widely into clinical practice. The NIH consensus development conferences may issue similar recommendations regarding the appropriate use and effectiveness of a new procedures in clinical use.

48. The heated debate in the American Association of Neurological Surgeons and the New England Journal of Medicine illustrates the difficulties a number of prominent physicians had accepting the EC/IC bypass trial results (112,113), as well as the importance of ensuring "clear definition and relative homogeneity of the patients to be randomized."

49. Inherent in his proposal is a fluid protocol that allows incremental changes in techniques.

50. Alternatively, Buxton—in a three-year evaluation of heart transplants in the United Kingdom—uses cross-sectional analyses to estimate changes in benefit and cost parameters over a longer time period than the study period directly allows (115).

51. The few clinical trials using sham operations clearly demonstrated that a strong placebo effect can be associated with these surgical interventions, thus underlining the importance of controls (119).

52. The OECD in general defines industrial companies with 11 percent of their turnover in R&D already as "research intensive" (111).

53. One furthermore should keep in mind that, whereas the success rates of NCEs are higher for 1970 cohorts than for earlier cohorts, at present 73 percent of NCEs initiating human testing are still discontinued before an NDA is submitted (63).

54. The number of drugs approved for the U.S. market averaged 36 NCEs per year between 1950 and 1960. A decline of 54 percent occurred in the early 1960s, after which the numbers fluctuated, averaging 14 NCEs per year through the end of the 1970s. Since the end of the 1970s, approval rates recovered somewhat (26 in 1985, 20 in 1986), though this recovery did not specifically take place in U.S.-originated but in foreign-owned approvals (30,31,125).

55. Notably, such benefits include the structural prevention of potentially unsafe and/or ineffective drugs; these basic premises on which the regulatory system is based are generally considered valuable. However, it is interesting that—in contrast to the medical device amendments—there is no legal mandate to encourage development and innovation, but only to assure the marketing of "safe and effective" drugs (124).

56. For example, getting a drug on the market one year earlier would reduce the average break-even point economically (i.e., where R&D costs equal revenues) by three to four years (128).

57. Grabowski (128) has determined that it would take 12 years of projected revenues at the present rate to achieve a real return on capital of 8 percent. A 10 percent real return would require 19 years of projected revenues at the present rate.

58. Furthermore, while the advantages for generic drugs can be reaped immediately, the advantages inherent in the law for innovative products can only be reaped further in the future (i.e., at the point where the patent term would have expired without the law).

59. Although a drug may continue to earn positive profits after the patent expiration date, under the pressure of generic competition the sales of a patent-expired product currently fall by 50 percent or more in the two or three years after patent expiry.

60. Furthermore, hospital formularies favor the lowest cost products, and the "Maximum Allowable Cost Program" reimburses Medicare patients only for the lowest cost product. In addition, international competition from Japan and Europe has increased. Recently the European Economic Community (EEC) introduced "the protection of the exclusive rights of the company that submits a file for regulatory approval. Files of new products, irrespective of the patent situation, will remain inaccessible to others for up to 10 years from the time the first EEC approval has been granted" (129).

61. "It is the purpose to encourage, to the extent consistent with the protection of the public health and safety and with ethical standards, the discovery and development of useful devices intended for human use and to that end to maintain optimum freedom for scientific investigators in their pursuit of that purpose" (Medical Device Ammendments 520, g(1)).

62. IDEs are devices under development which require FDA approval to initiate clinical evaluation in humans.

63. Consider, for example, the management of angina. The development of coronary artery bypass surgery and of beta-blockers were initiated at roughly the same time. The imbalance in assessment strategies, however, implies that the surgical option could undergo much more rapid diffusion than the pharmacological option, as beta-blockers were not as rapidly available to practicing physicians.

64. A subsequent study by Grabowski et al. (133) used a more sophisticated model, and found roughly similar results. As a measure of regulation they considered the average amount of NDA review time. Regarding research opportunities, they used changes in the productivity of pharmaceutical R&D in the United Kingdom during the 1960s as a control measure for changes in non-regulatory factors in the United States.

65. However, one should keep in mind that the four largest drug categories in the early 1960s—anti-infectives, analgesics, cardiovasculars, and psychopharmacologics—still remained the largest therapeutic categories in the early 1980s.

66. While, as mentioned above, assessing efficacy and safety may be more complex with psychopharmacological products, this is certainly not the case with anti-infectives. Furthermore, the NDA review times within the regulatory agency for these two categories were rather similar with regard to drugs in other therapeutic classes. In addition, the percentage of psychopharmacological drugs and anti-infectives first marketed abroad (under a different regulatory system) were also

roughly similar to the percentage first marketed abroad in other therapeutic classes. According to these measures, it appears that neither psychopharmacological products nor anti-infectives were regulated more stringently. The additional decline in these two categories, above other categories, therefore should be related to a number of non-regulatory factors, such as a potential decrease in research opportunities, or a potential increase in perceived risk of developing drugs in a specific area (for instance, a relationship between the decrease in tranquilizers and the thalidomide tragedy).

REFERENCES

1. Bernal JD. Science in History. Volume I–IV. Illustrated edition. Gretna, La.: Pelican Books, 1969.
2. Freeman C, Clark J, Soete L. Unemployment and Technical Innovation. London, 1982.
3. Rosenberg N. Inside the Black Box: Technology and Economics. New York: Cambridge University Press, 1982.
4. Landau R, Rosenberg N. The Positive Sum Strategy. Washington, D.C.: National Academy Press, 1986.
5. Casimir HBG. Haphazard Reality, Half a Century of Science. New York: Harper & Row Publishers, 1983.
6. Kline SJ, Rosenberg N. An overview of innovation. In Landau R, Rosenberg N (eds). The Positive Sum Strategy. Washington, D.C.: National Academy Press, 1986:275–306.
7. Mowery D, Rosenberg N. The influence of market demand upon innovation: A critical review of some recent empirical studies. Research Policy 1979;8:102–153.
8. Hillman BJ. Government health policy and the diffusion of new medical devices. Health Services Research 1986;21:681–711.
9. Fox RC. The cultural shaping of biomedical science and technology. A preface. International Journal of Technology Assessment in Health Care 1986;2:189–194.
10. Nelson RR, Winter SG. In search of useful theory of innovation. Research Policy 1977;6:36–76.
11. Greer AL. Adoption of medical technology: The hospital's three decision-systems. International Journal of Technology Assessment in Health Care 1985;1:669–680.
12. Cody E. France orders sale of new pill. Washington Post, 1988.
13. Liebenau J. Innovation in pharmaceuticals: Industrial R&D in the early 20th century. Research Policy 1985;14:179–187.
14. Felig P. Biomedical research in the industrial setting: Contrasts and similarities to academia. Journal of the American Medical Association 1987;258:2407–2409.
15. Thier SO. Public policy and private sector innovation. Keynote Address at the Pharmaceutical Manufacturers Association Meeting on America's Medical Research, Washington, D.C., November 1987.
16. Mansfield E, Rapoport J, Wagner S, Hamburger M. Research and innovation in the modern corporation. New York: W.W. Norton, 1971.
17. Cuatrecasas P. Contemporary Drug Development—Dilemmas. The Center for the Study of Drug Development Publication Series. New York: University of Rochester, 1983.

18. Spilker B. Multinational Drug Companies: Issues in Drug Discovery and Development. New York: Raven Press, 1989.

19. Maxwell RA. The state of the art of the science of drug discovery—an opinion. Drug Development Research 1984;4:380.

20. Wardell WM, Sheck LE. Is pharmaceutical innovation declining? In Lindgren B (ed). Pharmaceutical Economics. Stockholm: Swedish Institute for Health Economics, Liber Forlag, 1984:180–182.

21. Ahlquist RP. Study of adrenotropic receptors. American Journal of Physiology 1948;53:586–600.

22. Powell EE, Slater IH. Blocking of inhibitory adrenergic receptors by a dichloro analog of isoproterenol. Journal of Pharmacology and Experimental Therapeutics 1958:122:480–488.

23. Black JW, Stephenson JS. Pharmacology of a new adrenergic beta-receptor-blocking compound (nethalide). Lancet 1962;2:311–314.

24. Black JW, Crowther AF, Shanks RG, Smith LH, Dornhorst AC. A new adrenergic beta-receptor antagonist. Lancet 1964;1:1080–1081.

25. Nobel Committee, Stockholm, 1988.

26. Frishman WH. Clinical differences between beta-adrenergic agents: Implications for therapeutic substitution. American Heart Journal 1987;113:1190–1198.

27. van der Linden W. Pitfalls in randomized surgical trials. Surgery 1980;87:258–262.

28. Zbinden G, Flury-Roversi M. Significance of the LD-50 test for the toxicological evaluation of chemical substances. Archives of Toxicology 1981;47:77–99.

29. Zbinden G. Current trends in safety testing and toxicological research. Naturwisenschaften 1982;69:255–259.

30. Kaitin KI, Richard BW, Lasagna L. Trends in drug development: The 1985–86 new drug approvals. Journal of Clinical Pharmacology 1987;27:542–548.

31. Mattison N, Trimble AG, Lasagna L. New drug development in the United States, 1963 through 1984. Clinical Pharmacology and Therapeutics 1988;43:290–301.

32. Wardell WM, Sheck LE. Is pharmaceutical innovation declining? In Lindgren B (ed). Pharmaceutical Economics. Stockholm: Swedish Institute for Health Economics, Liber Forlag, 1984:180–182.

33. Barton Hutt P. Regulation in the United States. International Journal of Technology Assessment in Health Care 1986;2:619–628.

34. FDA Office of Planning and Evaluation. Assessment of the economic impact of revisions to regulations governing the submission of investigational new drug applications. Rockville, Md.: Food and Drug Administration, 1984.

35. Lasagna L, Bearn AG. Innovation and Acceleration in Clinical Drug Development. Roundtable 2: Early clinical trials—Phase I–IIA: Optimal designs for maximum information. New York: Raven Press, 1987, pp. 95–103.

36. Tucker SA, Blozan C, Coppinger P. The outcome of research on new molecular entities commencing clinical research in the years 1976–1978. Office of Planning and Evaluation, study 77. Rockville, Md.: Food and Drug Administration, 1988.

37. Nightingale SL. Drug regulation and policy formulation. Milbank Memorial Fund Quarterly 1981;3:412–444.

38. Eschbach JW. Presentation at the Institute of Medicine. The workshop New Biology: Impact on Drug Development. Washington, D.C.: National Academy Press, 1989.

39. Doyle AE. Biologic end-points as surrogates for clinical outcomes. In Lasagna L, Bearn AG (eds). Innovation and Acceleration in Clinical Drug Development. New York: Raven Press, 1987:117–123.

40. Bergner M. Quality of Life, Health Status, and Clinical Research. In Lohr KN (ed). Advances in Health Status Assessment: Conference Procedings. Medical Care 1989; 27:148–156.

41. General Accounting Office. FDA Drug Approval—a lengthy process that delays the availability of important new drugs. Hearings before the Subcommittee on Science, Research, and Technology. May 1980.

42. Moses LE. Randomized Clinical Trials. In Assessing Medical Technologies. Institute of Medicine. Washington, D.C.: National Academy Press, 1985:73–80.

43. Chalmers TC. The clinical trial. Milbank Memorial Fund Quarterly 1981;59:324–339.

44. Young FE, Norris JA, Levitt JA et al. The FDA's new procedures for the use of investigational drugs in treatment. Journal of the American Medical Association 1988;259:2267–2270.

45. Wardell WM, Tsianco MC, Anaveliar SN, Dans HT. Postmarketing surveillance of new drugs II. Case Studies. Journal of Clinical Pharmacology 1979;19:169–184.

46. Lasagna L. Techniques for ADR reporting. Detection and prevention of adverse drug reactions. Stockholm: Almquist G. Wichsell International, 1984:146–151.

47. Wiener H. Problems in the assessment of side effects of new drugs. New York: Pfizer Pharmaceuticals, internal document.

48. McKinlay SM. Experimentation in human populations. Milbank Memorial Fund Quarterly 1981;59:308–323.

49. FDA Consumer Special Report. From test tube to patient: New drug development in the U.S. Rockville, Md.: Food and Drug Administration, January 1988.

50. FDA Office of Planning and Evaluation. Final regulatory impact analysis of changes to regulations governing the submission and review of new drug applications. Part 314, Title 21. Rockville, Md.: Food and Drug Administration, August 1983.

51. Maynard A, Hartley K. The regulation of the pharmaceutical industry. In Lindgren B (ed). Pharmaceutical Economics. Stockholm: Swedish Institute for Health Economics, Liber Forlag, 1984:123–137.

52. Medica-Pharmaceutical Forum. Clinical Trials. London: Royal Society of Medicine Services, 1987.

53. Jones JK. Regulatory use of adverse drug reactions. Stockholm: Skandia International Symposia, Almquist G. Wichsell International, 1984:203–214.

54. Joint Commission on Prescription Drug Use. Final Report. Washington, D.C.: Government Printing Office, April 1980.

55. Borden EK, Lee JG. A methodological study of post-marketing drug evaluation using a pharmacy-based approach. Journal of Chronic Diseases 1982;35:803–816.

56. Inman WHW. Drug Surveillance Research Unit. Letter from the director. University of Southampton. PEM News 1983;N1.

57. Wennberg JE, Roos N, Sola L, Schori A, Jaffe R. Use of claims data systems to evaluate health care outcomes. Journal of the American Medical Association 1987:257:933–936.

58. Mattison N, Richard BW. Postapproval research requested by the FDA at the time

of NCE approval, 1970–1984. Drug Information Journal 1987;21:309–329.

59. Levy RI, Sondik EJ. The management of biomedical research: An example for heart, lung, blood diseases. In Roberts EB, Levy RI, Finestein SW, Moskowitz J, Sondik EJ. Biomedical Innovation. Cambridge: Massachusetts Institute of Technology Press, 1981.

60. Feinstein AR. Clinical Biostatistics. St. Louis: Mosby, 1977.

61. Eden M. The engineering-industrial accord: Inventing the technology of health care. In Reiser SJ, Anbar M (eds). The Machine at the Bedside. New York: Cambridge University Press, 1984.

62. Thomas LJ. Federal support of medical device innovation. In Ekelman K (ed). New Medical Devices: Innovation, Development, and Use. Washington, D.C., National Academy Press, 1988:59, 61.

63. National Research Council. Directions in Engineering Research. An Assessment of Opportunities and Needs. Washington, D.C.: National Academy Press, 1987: 84–85.

64. Office of Technology Assessment. Federal policies and the medical devices industry, October 1984. Washington, D.C., 1988.

65. Pollard MR, Persinger GS. Investment in health care innovation. Health Affairs 1987;Summer:93–100.

66. U.S. Department of Commerce, Bureau of Industrial Economics. U.S. Industrial Outlook. Washington, D.C., 1983.

67. Spilker B. Planning studies to evaluate medical devices. In Guide to Planning and Managing Multiple Clinical Studies. New York: Raven Press, 1987.

68. Roberts EB. Technological innovation and medical device innovation. In Ekelman K (ed). New Medical Devices: Innovation, Development, and Use. Washington, D.C.: National Academy Press, 1988.

69. von Hippel E. The dominant role of users in the scientific instrument innovation process. Research Policy 1976;3:212–239.

70. von Hippel E, Finkelstein S. Product designs which encourage or discourage related innovations by users: An analysis of innovation in automatic clinical chemistry analyzers. Working paper. Sloan School of Management. Cambridge: Massachusetts Institute of Technology, 1978.

71. Whitehead EC. Development of technicians auto analyzer. In Ekelman K (ed). New Medical Devices: Innovation, Development and Use. Washington, D.C., National Academy Press, 1988.

72. Shaw BF. The role of the interaction between the manufacturer and the user in the technological innovation process. Ph.D. dissertation. Sussex, U.K., 1987.

73. Allen TJ. Communication Networks in R&D Laboratories. R&D Management 1970;1:14–21.

74. Roberts EB, Peters D. Commercial innovation from university faculty. Research Policy 1981;2:108–126.

75. Melmon KL. Strategic planning and the transfer of technology to clinical medicine. Presented to the Stanford Alumni Association, North Carolina, March 17, 1989.

76. Office of Planning and Evaluation. Pre-amendment medical device safety and efficacy testing. Rockville, Md.: Food and Drug Administration, October 1982.

77. Arthur D. Little. Medical device safety and efficacy testing PB 83-105-031; PB 83-105-049; PB 82-113-036.

78. Food, Drug, and Cosmetics Act, Section 501 to 521.
79. Kennedy RS. Clinical investigations with medical devices: New rules. Journal of the American Medical Association 1981;245:2053–2054.
80. Food and Drug Administration. The Code of Federal Regulations. Section 860.3.
81. Kessler DA, Pape SM, Sundwall DN. The federal regulation of medical devices. New England Journal of Medicine 1987:317:357–365.
82. General Accounting Office. Medical Devices—FDA's 510(k) operations could be improved. August 1988.
83. IDE regulations. 45 Federal Register 3732, 1980.
84. Blozan CF, Gieser NC, Tucker SA. A profile of investigational device exemption applications. OPE study 76. Rockville, Md.: Food and Drug Administration, November 1987.
85. Fineberg HV, Bauman R, Susman M. Computerized cranial tomography: Effect on diagnostic and therapeutic plans. Journal of the American Medical Association 1977;238:224–230.
86. Horwitz RI, Feinstein AR, Crede WB, Clemens JD. Does technology work? Judging the validity of clinical evidence. In Reiser SJ, Anbar M (eds). The Machine at the Bedside. New York: Cambridge University Press, 1984:193–208.
87. McNeil BJ, Keeler E, Adelstein SJ. Primer on certain elements of decision making. New England Journal of Medicine 1975;293:211–215.
88. Friedman PJ. The early evaluation of MR imaging. American Journal of Radiology 1988;151:860–861.
89. Schwartz JS. Evaluating diagnostic technologies. In Assessing Medical Technologies. Institute of Medicine. Washington, D.C.: National Academy Press, 1985:80–89.
90. Barton Hutt P. Medical device regulation: Reasonable workable. Legal Times Washington, May 1980.
91. Russel LB. The Diffusion of New Hospital Technologies in the United States. International Journal of Health Services 1976;4:557–580.
92. Anderson GF, Steinberg E. To buy or not to buy technology: Acquisition under prospective payment. New England Journal of Medicine 1984;311:182–185.
93. Moxley JH. How trends will interact: The perspective of the hospital. In Ekelman K (ed). New Medical Devices: Innovation, Development, and Use. Washington, D.C.: National Academy Press, 1988:127–137.
94. Altman SM. Impact of the changing medical payment system in technological innovation and utilization. In Ekelman K (ed). New Medical Devices: Innovation, Development and Use. Washington, D.C.: National Academy Press, 1988:93–103.
95. National Advisory Council on Health Care Technology Assessment. The Medicare Coverage Process. Office of the Assistant Secretary for Health, Department of Health and Human Services, September 1988.
96. Carr SW, Jones JH. Drug epidemiology data bases applicable to medical device monitoring. Medical Device Data Base Conference, Washington D.C., American Medical Association, October 1983.
97. Green SB, Byar DP. Using observational data from registries to compare treatments: The fallacy of omnimetrics. Statistics in Medicine 1984;3:361–370.
98. Shephard D, Durch JS. International comparison of resource allocation in health sciences: An analysis of expenditures on biomedical research in 19 industrialized

countries. Supported by the Fogarty International Center, National Institutes of Health. Harvard School of Public Health, 1985.

99. Swazey, JP, Fox RC. The clinical moratorium. In Fox RC. Essays in Medical Sociology. New York: Wiley-Interscience, 1974:325–363.

100. Sladek JR, Shoulson I. Neural transplantation: A call for patience rather than patients. Science 1988;240:1386–1388.

101. Fox RC, Swazey J. The Courage to Fail: A Social View of Organ Transplants and Dialysis. Chicago: University of Chicago Press, 1974.

102. Comroe JH, Dripps RD. Scientific basis for the support of biomedical science. In Roberts EB, Levy RI, Finestein SW, Moskowitz J, Sondik EJ: Biomedical Innovation. Cambridge: MIT Press, 1981.

103. Moore FD. Therapeutic innovation: Ethical boundaries in the initial clinical trials of new drugs and surgical procedures. Daedalus 1969;Spring:502–522.

104. Bergkamp L. American IRBs and Dutch Research Ethics Committees: How they compare. IRB: A Review of Human Subjects Research. Hastings Center 1988;10:1–6.

105. Barnes BA. Discarded operations: Surgical innovation by trial and error. In Bunker JP, Barnes BA, Mosteller F (eds). Costs, Risks and Benefits of Surgery. Oxford University Press, 1977:109–123.

106. Bunker JP, Barnes BA, Mosteller F (eds). Costs, Risks and Benefits of Surgery. Oxford University Press, 1977.

107. Bunker JP, Hinkley D, McDermott WV. Surgical innovation and its evaluation. Science 1978;200:937–941.

108. Eddy DM, Billings J. The quality of medical evidence: Implications for quality of care. Health Affairs 1988;Spring:20–32.

109. Wennberg JE. Improving the medical decision making process. Health Affairs 1988;Spring:99–106.

110. Gilbert JP, McPeek B, Mosteller F. Statistics and ethics in surgery and anesthesia. Science 1977;198:684–689.

111. Office of Economic Cooperation and Development (OECD). Science and technology indicators. No.2: R&D, Invention and Competitiveness. Paris, March 1986.

112. EC/IC Bypass Study Group. Failure of extracranial-intracranial arterial bypass to reduce the risk of ischemic stroke. New England Journal of Medicine 1985;313:1191–1200.

113. EC/IC Bypass Study Group. Are the Results of the Extracranial-Intracranial Bypass Trial Generalizable? New England Journal of Medicine 1987;13:820–824.

114. Chalmers TC. Randomization and coronary artery surgery. Annals of Thoracic Surgery 1972;14:323–327.

115. Buxton M. Problems in the economic appraisal of new health technology: The evaluation of heart transplants in the United Kingdom. In Drummond MF (ed). Economic Appraisal of Health Technology in the European Community. Oxford Medical Publications, 1987.

116. Feinstein AR. An additional basic science for clinical medicine: II. The limitations of randomized trials. Annals of Internal Medicine 1983;49:544–550.

117. Bonchek LI. The role of the randomized clinical trial in the evaluation of new operations. Surgical Clinics of North America 1982;62:761–769.

118. Bonchek LI. Are randomized trials appropriate for evaluating new operations? New England Journal of Medicine 1979;301:44–45.

119. Dimond EG, Kittle CF, Crockett JE. Comparison of internal mammary artery ligation and sham operation for angina pectoris. American Journal of Cardiology 1960;5:483–486.

120. Hlatky MA, Lee KL, Harrel FE, Califf RM, Pryor DB, Marck DB, Rosatti RA. Tying clinical research to patient care by use of an observational database. Statistics in Medicine 1984;3:375–384.

121. Roos LL et al. Computers to identify complications after surgery. American Journal of Public Health 1985;75:1288–1294.

122. Kaye HL. The biological revolution and its cultural context. International Journal of Technology Assessment in Health Care 1986;2:275–284.

123. Wiggins SN. The cost of developing a new drug. Pharmaceutical Manufacturers Association, Washington, D.C., June 1987.

124. Laubach GB. Federal regulation and pharmaceutical innovation. In Levin A (ed). Regulating Health Care: The Structure for Control. Proceedings of Political Science 1980;3:64–80.

125. May MS, Wardell WM, Lasagna L. New drug development during and after a period of regulatory change: Clinical research activity of major United States pharmaceutical firms, 1958 to 1979. Clinical Pharmacology and Therapeutics 1983;33:691–700.

126. Pharmaceutical Manufacturers Association. Update on biotechnology products in development. Washington, D.C., July 1988.

127. Temin P. Taking Your Medicine: Drug Regulation in the United States. Cambridge, Mass.: Harvard University Press, 1980.

128. Grabowski HG. Health Care Cost Containment and Pharmaceutical Innovation. Boston: Center for the Study of Drug Development, 1986. Reprint RS S707.

129. Wiedhaup K. View of contraceptive development. Presentation for the National Research Council, Washington, D.C., March 1988.

130. Read JL, Campbell PM. Health care innovation: A progress report. Health Affairs. 1988;Summer:174–185.

131. Peltzman S. An evaluation of consumer protection regulation: The 1962 drug amendment. Journal of Political Economy 1973;81:1049–91.

132. Baily MN. Research and development costs and returns: The U.S. pharmaceutical industry. Journal of Political Economy 1972;80:78–85.

133. Grabowski HG, Vernon J, Thomas L. Estimating the effects of regulation on innovation: An international comparative analysis of the pharmaceutical industry. Journal of Law and Economics 1978;21:1–32.

134. Wiggins SN. The effect of U.S. pharmaceutical regulations on new introductions. In Lindgren B (ed). Pharmaceutical Economics. Stockholm: Swedish Institute for Health Economics, Liber Forlag, 1984:191–205, 195–201.

135. Wardell WM. Introduction of new drugs in the United States and Great Britain: An international comparison. Clinical Pharmacology and Therapeutics 1973; 14:773–790.

136. Wardell WM. Therapeutic implications of the drug lag. Clinical Pharmacology and Therapeutics 1974;15:73–96.

137. Wardell WM. The drug lag revisited: Comparison by therapeutic area of drugs marketed in the United States and Great Britain from 1972 through 1976. Clinical Pharmacology and Therapeutics 1978;24:499–527.

138. Bakke OM, Wardell WM, Lasagna L. Drug discontinuations in the United

Kingdom and the U.S., 1964 to 1983: Issues of safety. Clinical Pharmacology and Therapeutics 1984;35:559–567.

139. Hass AE, Portable DP, Grossman RE. New Drug Introductions, Discontinuations and Safety Issues in the United States and the United Kingdom: 1960–1982. OPE (FDA) study 68.

140. Berlin H, Jonsson B. International dissemination of new drugs: A comparative study of six countries. Managerial and Decision Economics 1986;7:235–242.

Appendix B

Workshop Agenda

**Improving the Translation of Research Findings into Clinical Practice:
I. The Potential and Problems of Modern Methods of Clinical
   Investigation**

Wednesday, May 3, 1989

8:00 a.m.	*Registration and Continental Breakfast*
8:30 a.m.	Welcome and Opening Remarks
	Samuel Thier, *President*, Institute of Medicine Gerald Laubach, *Chair*, Committee on Technological Innovation in Medicine
Session One:	**Setting the Stage**
	Keynote Address 8:45 a.m. Technological Innovation and Evaluation in Medicine Samuel Thier, Institute of Medicine
Session Two:	**Outcomes and Evaluative Research** *Moderator:* Paul Parkman, Food and Drug Administration

9:15 a.m.	The Selection of Endpoints in Evaluative Research John Bunker, Stanford University
9:45 a.m.	Advances in Health Status Measurement: The Potential to Improve Experimental and Non-Experimental Data Collection Marilyn Bergner, Johns Hopkins University
10:15 a.m.	General Discussion
10:45 a.m.	*Break*
Session Three:	**Modern Epidemiologic Methods for Obtaining Primary Evidence** *Moderator:* Paul Stolley, University of Pennsylvania
11:00 a.m.	What Is Outcomes Research? John Wennberg, Dartmouth College
11:45 a.m.	Strengths and Weaknesses of Health Insurance Data Systems for Assessing Outcomes Leslie Roos and Noralou Roos, University of Manitoba, Canada
12:15 p.m.	General Discussion
1:00 p.m.	*Lunch*
2:00 p.m.	Prescription-Event Monitoring: An Example of Total Population Post-Marketing Drug Surveillance William Inman, Drug Safety Research Unit, United Kingdom Discussant: Brian Strom, University of Pennsylvania
2:30 p.m.	General Discussion
Session Four:	**Modern Methods to Synthesize Existing Evidence** *Moderator:* Frederick Mosteller, Harvard University
3:00 p.m.	The Value of Modern Methods of Decision Analysis Albert Mulley, Massachusetts General Hospital

3:30 p.m.	The Value of Modern Methods of Meta-Analysis Stephen Thacker, Center for Environmental Health and Injury Control, Centers for Disease Control
4:00 p.m.	A Bayesian Approach to Clinical Evaluation David Eddy, Duke University
4:30 p.m.	General Discussion
5:30 p.m.	*Adjourn and Reception*
6:15 p.m.	*Dinner*

Thursday, May 4, 1989

8:30 a.m.	*Continental Breakfast*
Session Five:	**Modern Methods of Clinical Evaluation: What Are the Challenges and Consequences for Technological Innovation in Medicine?**
	Keynote Address 9:15 a.m. Can We Improve the Transfer of Research Findings Into Clinical Practice Through Modern Methods of Evaluation? David Eddy, Duke University
10:00 a.m.	*Break*
10:15 a.m.	**Roundtable Discussion (A)** *Moderator:* Harvey Fineberg, Harvard University *Panel Members:* David Eddy, Duke University Alvan Feinstein, Yale University Robert Levy, Sandoz Research Institute Robert Temple, Food and Drug Administration Salim Yusuf, National Heart, Lung, and Blood Institute
11:45 a.m.	*Lunch*
12:45 p.m.	Factors That Influence the Utilization of Modern Evaluative Methods Kenneth Melmon, Stanford University

1:30 p.m.   **Roundtable Discussion (B)**
Moderator: Charles Sanders, Squibb
Panel Members:
Susan Bartlett Foote, University of California, Berkeley
Jere Goyan, University of California, San Francisco
Ben Holmes, Hewlett-Packard
William Hubbard, Council on Health Care Technology,
Institute of Medicine
Kenneth Melmon, Stanford University
Stephen Sherwin, Genentech
M. Roy Schwarz, American Medical Association

3:00 p.m.   Summary of the Meeting
Gerald Laubach, Chair, Committee on Technological
Innovation in Medicine

3:15 p.m.   *Adjourn*

Appendix C

Contributors

MARILYN BERGNER is professor of health policy and management at the Johns Hopkins School of Hygiene and Public Health. She also is a member of the Health Services Research and Development Center and the Program in Medical Technology and Practice Assessment of Johns Hopkins. Before joining Johns Hopkins, Dr. Bergner was a faculty member at the University of Washington. With her colleagues she developed the Sickness Impact Profile, a widely used health status measure that assesses health-related behavioral dysfunction. Dr. Bergner has written extensively in the area of health status measurement. She received her Ph.D. from Columbia University.

THOMAS A. BUBOLZ has been on the faculty in community and family medicine at Dartmouth Medical School since 1986. He is the designer and administrator of a 300-million record data management system at Dartmouth that supports studies in the epidemiology of health care utilization and outcomes for various surgical and medical therapies. Dr. Bubolz is managing the development of analytic software for small-area and outcomes research. His current research is on the application of claims data to the assessment of rural-urban differences in health care utilization and outcomes. Dr. Bubolz was on the faculty in statistics at Iowa State University from 1974 to 1985, where he taught undergraduate and graduate courses in statistical computing and data analysis and supervised a computer applications development group. He coauthored the RELIABILITY procedure in SPSSX, a program widely used for evaluating multi-item scales in behavioral and psychometric research. Dr. Bubolz has collaborated with associations and state agencies in Iowa on small-area studies of health care utilization.

JOHN P. BUNKER is professor emeritus at Stanford University and a visiting fellow at the King's Fund Centre for Health Services Development in London. At Stanford he was professor and chairman of the Department of Anesthesia from 1960 to 1972 and more recently professor of health research and policy, director of the program in Health Services Research, and chairman of the Council of the Consortium on Health Research and Policy. He was chairman of the National Research Council Committee on the National Halothane Study and senior editor of its report published in 1969. As visiting professor of preventive and social medicine at Harvard Medical School, he chaired the surgical study group and its parent seminar in health and medicine. The proceedings of the surgical study group, for which he was senior editor, were published in 1977 as *Costs, Risks, and Benefits of Surgery*. His most recent publication is *Pathways to Health: The Role of Social Factors*, which he edited with Deanna S. Gomby and Barbara H. Kehrer. Together with Frederick Mosteller he currently heads a newly formed program of research, Pathways to Health: The Role of Medical Care. Dr. Bunker is former chairman of the Health Services Research Study Section of the National Center for Health Services Research. He is a graduate of Harvard College and Harvard Medical School.

DAVID M. EDDY is the J. Alexander McMahon Professor of Health Policy and Management at Duke University. He received his M.D. degree from the University of Virginia. After two years of residency in cardiovascular surgery at Stanford, he left clinical practice and received a Ph.D. in engineering-economic systems (applied mathematics) at Stanford. After serving on the faculty at Stanford as a professor of engineering and medicine, he went to Duke University in 1981 to set up the Center for Health Policy Research and Education. Dr. Eddy's research has been to develop and apply methods for evaluating health practices and designing practice policies. He has developed policies and related guidlines for organizations such as the American Cancer Society, National Cancer Institute, World Health Organization, the Office of Technology Assessment, the Blue Cross and Blue Shield Association, the Council of Medical Specialty Societies, and the American Medical Association. His mathematical model of cancer screening was awarded the Lanchester Prize, the top award in the field of operations research. He has recently completed a book that describes a new set of statistical methods for synthesizing evidence to estimate the effect of medical interventions on health outcomes. Dr. Eddy serves on the Board of Mathematics of the National Academy of Sciences and is a member of the Institute of Medicine.

ELLIOTT S. FISHER received his medical degree from Harvard. He completed residency training in internal medicine and public health at the University of Washington, where he was also a fellow in the Robert Wood Johnson Clinical Scholars Program. In Washington State he was active in health policy, helping develop a pilot state-funded health insurance program for the uninsured. Since

1986 Dr. Fisher has been on the faculty at Dartmouth Medical School and on the staff of the Veterans Administration (VA) hospital in White River Junction. He has worked with both Medicare and VA health care data bases and is currently the director of a project to develop claims-based methods for evaluating both utilization patterns and outcomes of care within the northeast region of the VA.

ANNETINE C. GELIJNS is international fellow at the Institute of Medicine and the principal staff officer for the IOM Committee on Technological Innovation in Medicine. Before joining the IOM, she was senior researcher for the Project on Future Health Care Technology cosponsored by the European office of the World Health Organization and the Dutch government. From 1983 to 1985, Ms. Gelijns worked for the Steering Committee on Future Health Scenarios, where she helped develop models for long-term health planning in the areas of cancer, cardiovascular disease, and aging. At the time, she had a joint appointment with the Staff Bureau for Health Policy Development, the Department of Health, the Netherlands. Ms. Gelijns has been a consultant to various national and international organizations, including the World Health Organization, the Organization for Economic Cooperation and Development, and the Dutch Health Council. In 1983 she received her LL.M. degree from the University of Leyden. Currently she is writing her Ph.D. dissertation on medical innovation for the University of Amsterdam. She received the Querido Award in support of her doctoral work from the Netherlands Praeventiefonds (Dutch Fund for Disease Prevention).

VIC HASSELBLAD is research associate professor at the Center for Health Policy Research and Education at Duke University. He received an M.S. degree in mathematical statistics from the University of Washington and a Ph.D. in biostatistics from the University of California, Los Angeles. Dr. Hasselblad then joined the U.S. government biometric group, which eventually became part of the Environmental Protection Agency. As a member of that organization, he was responsible for the design, conduct, and analysis of empirical epidemiological and toxicological studies, as well as the development of new methods for analyzing epidemiological and toxicological problems. In 1982, Dr. Hasselblad was given the Environmental Protection Agency's Scientific and Technology Achievement Award for his work, and in 1985 he joined the Center for Health Policy Research and Education. His main research interest is in developing statistical methods for evaluating health technologies. This work has culminated in the coauthorship of a recent book on statistical methods for synthesizing evidence. He has published widely in the epidemiological, statistical, and medical literature on health and methodological topics.

WILLIAM H. W. INMAN has been responsible for developing both national systems for monitoring drug safety in the United Kingdom. In 1964, following the thalidomide tragedy, he was invited by Sir Derrick Dunlop to develop the yellow card system and, as principal medical officer in the Department of Health, was medical assessor of adverse reactions for the Committee on Safety of Drugs. In 1980 Dr. Inman was seconded to the University of Southampton to establish the independent Drug Safety Research Unit and in 1984 was appointed to the first chair in pharmacoepidemiology to be established in the United Kingdom. Dr. Inman received his M.A., M.B., and B.Chir. at Cambridge University, and in 1981 he became a fellow of the Royal College of Physicians.

GERALD D. LAUBACH is president of Pfizer, Inc., and chair of the Institute of Medicine (IOM) Committee on Technological Innovation in Medicine. Dr. Laubach is a research chemist by training and served as a laboratory scientist in his early years at Pfizer. He is a member of the IOM and the National Academy of Engineering and serves on the IOM Council on Health Care Technology. His current activities also include membership on the executive committee of the Council on Competitiveness (successor group to the President's Commission on Industrial Competitiveness), the boards of the Food and Drug Law Institute, the Carnegie Institution of Washington, and the National Committee for Quality Health Care, and the Corporation Committee for Sponsored Research at the Massachusetts Institute of Technology and directorships of CIGNA Corporation of Philadephia and the Millipore Corporation of Bedford, Massachusetts. Previously, Dr. Laubach served as chair of the Pharmaceutical Manufacturers Association from 1977 to 1978 and as a board member until April 1989. Dr. Laubach holds a B.A. from the University of Pennsylvania and a Ph.D. in organic chemistry from the Massachusetts Institute of Technology.

KENNETH L. MELMON received his undergraduate and medical training at Stanford and the University of California Medical Center, respectively. He trained for three years at the National Institutes of Health in the Experimental Therapeutics Branch of the National Heart Institute. After completing a final year of medical training as a chief resident at the University of Washington King County Hospital, Dr. Melmon joined the medical faculty at the University of California at San Francisco, where he instituted one of the first programs for research and training in clinical pharmacology. His research has focused on the pharmacology of the immune response. Dr. Melmon served as the chairperson of the Commission on Prescription Drug Use (1976-1980) where he became familiar with the methodology that might be used for detecting the effects of marketed drugs. Since that period he has contributed to the literature regarding the need to systematically detect the effects of marketed drugs and, secondarily, of devices and procedures. He joined the Stanford Medical School faculty in 1978 as chair of the Department of Medicine. Dr. Melmon presently serves as professor of medicine and pharmacology and associate chair of the Department of Medicine at Stanford University School of Medicine.

ALBERT G. MULLEY, JR., is associate professor of medicine and associate professor of health policy at Harvard Medical School and chief of the General Internal Medicine Unit at Massachusetts General Hospital. After receiving degrees in medicine and public policy from Harvard, he completed his residency training in internal medicine at Massachusetts General Hospital. He is author and editor of the text *Primary Care Medicine* and of many articles in the medical and health services research literature. Dr. Mulley's research has included the evaluation of medical intensive care and the cost effectiveness of prevention strategies and other common clinical practices. Recent work has focused on the use of decision analysis, outcomes research, and preference assessment methods to distinguish between warranted and unwarranted variations in clinical practices. In 1981 he was among the first general internists to receive the Henry J. Kaiser Family Foundation Faculty Scholar Award. He is a member of the Clinical Efficacy Assessment Subcommittee of the American College of Physicians and the Institute of Medicine Medicare Quality Assurance Committee.

LESLIE L. ROOS graduated from Stanford University and received his doctoral degree in political science from the Massachusetts Institute of Technology. Before coming to the University of Manitoba in 1973, he held faculty positions at Brandeis, Northwestern, and Indiana universities. He has held a National Health Scientist Award from the Research Programs Directorate, Health and Welfare, Canada, since 1982. Dr. Roos is a member of the Department of Community Health Sciences (Faculty of Medicine) and the Department of Business Administration (Faculty of Management) at the University of Manitoba. He is an associate of the Canadian Institute for Advanced Research.

NORALOU P. ROOS graduated from Stanford University and received her doctoral degree in political science from the Massachusetts Institute of Technology. Before coming to the University of Manitoba in 1973, she taught at MIT and at Northwestern University. She has held a National Health Scientist Award from the Research Programs Directorate, Health and Welfare, Canada, since 1975. Dr. Roos teaches in the Department of Community Health Sciences (Faculty of Medicine) at the University of Manitoba. She is an associate of the Canadian Institute for Advanced Research.

ROSS D. SHACHTER received an S.B. from the Massachusetts Institute of Technology and M.S. and Ph.D. degrees in operations research from the University of California, Berkeley. Since 1982 he has been an assistant professor in the Department of Engineering-Economic Systems at Stanford University and a participating faculty member in the Section on Medical Informatics. His research involves decision making under uncertainty, with emphasis on medical decision making and on the representation and analysis of decision models with influence diagrams. During the academic years 1986-1988 Dr. Shachter was a visiting professor at the Center for Health Policy Research and Education at Duke University, where he developed interactive analytical tools to assist in medical technology assessment. He is an active participant and organizer of the Workshops on Uncertainty in Artificial Intelligence and an officer of the Operations Research Society's Special Interest Group on Decision Analysis.

STEPHEN B. THACKER is currently director of the Epidemiology Program Office, Centers for Disease Control (CDC). Dr. Thacker came to the CDC in 1976 and became the first director of the Division of Surveillance and Epidemiologic Studies in the CDC Epidemiology Program Office. After chairing the committee that developed the first comprehensive CDC plan for public health surveillance, he was chosen to be the assistant director for science, Center for Environmental Health and Injury Control. Dr. Thacker received his undergraduate degree at Princeton University and his M.D. from the Mount Sinai School of Medicine in 1973. He completed residency training in family medicine at the Duke University School of Medicine. At Duke, Dr. Thacker was also a Robert Wood Johnson clinical scholar. In 1984, Dr. Thacker was awarded an M.Sc. in epidemiology from the London School of Hygiene and Tropical Medicine. Dr. Thacker currently holds appointments at both the Emory University School of Medicine and Mount Sinai School of Medicine. Dr. Thacker has published in a broad range of fields in epidemiology, including public health surveillance, infectious disease, and technology assessment. He has written papers on electronic fetal monitoring, ultrasound, methodologies for surveillance of medical technologies, and related areas.

SAMUEL O. THIER is president of the Institute of Medicine. Dr. Thier's previous appointments include Sterling Professor and chair of the Department of Medicine at Yale University School of Medicine, vice chair and professor of medicine at the University of Pennsylvania Medical School, and chief of the renal unit and assistant professor of medicine at Harvard Medical School. Dr. Thier did research at the National Institutes of Health from 1962 to 1964 and served on the director's advisory committee from 1980 to 1984. He is the author of numerous articles on renal physiology, inherited diseases of the kidney, and kidney stones and is coauthor of a textbook on pathophysiology. Dr. Thier has served as president of the American College of Physicians and as chair of the American Board of Internal Medicine. He received his undergraduate degree from Cornell University and his M.D. degree from the State University of New York at Syracuse.

JOHN E. WENNBERG is director of the Center for the Evaluative Clinical Sciences and professor of epidemiology at Dartmouth Medical School. He is a graduate of Stanford University and McGill Medical School, Montreal. Dr. Wennberg serves on a number of national committees, including the Health

Sciences Policy Board for the Institute of Medicine, the Accreditation Project Steering Committee for the Joint Commission, and the Board of Directors of the Collaborating Center for Small Area Analysis, University of Copenhagen, Denmark. Dr. Wennberg is the author of numerous publications and is particularly well known for his leading research in small-area variations in health care. He is currently principal investigator for the Prostate Assessment Team established under a new U.S. government program for outcomes research.

Index